Marco Beltrame

O3-DPACS: an open source PACS solution for the O3 Consortium project

Marco Beltrame

O3-DPACS: an open source PACS solution for the O3 Consortium project

The experience of designing and deploying a critical open source system

VDM Verlag Dr. Müller

Impressum/Imprint (nur für Deutschland/ only for Germany)

Bibliografische Information der Deutschen Nationalbibliothek: Die Deutsche Nationalbibliothek verzeichnet diese Publikation in der Deutschen Nationalbibliografie; detaillierte bibliografische Daten sind im Internet über http://dnb.d-nb.de abrufbar.

Alle in diesem Buch genannten Marken und Produktnamen unterliegen warenzeichen-, marken- oder patentrechtlichem Schutz bzw. sind Warenzeichen oder eingetragene Warenzeichen der jeweiligen Inhaber. Die Wiedergabe von Marken, Produktnamen, Gebrauchsnamen, Handelsnamen, Warenbezeichnungen u.s.w. in diesem Werk berechtigt auch ohne besondere Kennzeichnung nicht zu der Annahme, dass solche Namen im Sinne der Warenzeichen- und Markenschutzgesetzgebung als frei zu betrachten wären und daher von jedermann benutzt werden dürften.

Coverbild: www.purestockx.com

Verlag: VDM Verlag Dr. Müller Aktiengesellschaft & Co. KG
Dudweiler Landstr. 99, 66123 Saarbrücken, Deutschland
Telefon +49 681 9100-698, Telefax +49 681 9100-988, Email: info@vdm-verlag.de
Zugl.: Trieste, University Of Trieste, Diss. 2008

Herstellung in Deutschland:
Schaltungsdienst Lange o.H.G., Berlin
Books on Demand GmbH, Norderstedt
Reha GmbH, Saarbrücken
Amazon Distribution GmbH, Leipzig
ISBN: 978-3-639-17521-9

Imprint (only for USA, GB)

Bibliographic information published by the Deutsche Nationalbibliothek: The Deutsche Nationalbibliothek lists this publication in the Deutsche Nationalbibliografie; detailed bibliographic data are available in the Internet at http://dnb.d-nb.de.

Any brand names and product names mentioned in this book are subject to trademark, brand or patent protection and are trademarks or registered trademarks of their respective holders. The use of brand names, product names, common names, trade names, product descriptions etc. even without a particular marking in this works is in no way to be construed to mean that such names may be regarded as unrestricted in respect of trademark and brand protection legislation and could thus be used by anyone.

Cover image: www.purestockx.com

Publisher:
VDM Verlag Dr. Müller Aktiengesellschaft & Co. KG
Dudweiler Landstr. 99, 66123 Saarbrücken, Germany
Phone +49 681 9100-698, Fax +49 681 9100-988, Email: info@vdm-publishing.com
Trieste, University Of Trieste, Diss. 2008

Printed in the U.S.A.
Printed in the U.K. by (see last page)
ISBN: 978-3-639-17521-9

Introduction

The student started his work towards the PhD. in 2005, joining the Bioengineering and ICT group of the University of Trieste. The core research of the group was in the *e-health* area and the student approached it with the project to design server solution for the integration of biomedical data in any environment.

During the first year he studied several integration techniques and practiced the design and architecture of software applications, facing the first of two IHE Connectathons. In this period, it was easy to understand the need for new solutions and it the study about which characteristics the new solutions should have started.

After having explored the field of *m-health* (mobile health, the use of portable and mobile devices for *e-health*) and the integration of documents in the *patient electronic health record*, the student supported the decision, taken by the group, that a complete model for new technology application in *e-health* should be proposed.

Therefore, the student contributed in the creation and definition of O3 Consortium project, a project started by the Higher Education in Clinical Engineering of University of Trieste to realize that model. The project defined a development model, a support model and a business model. Moreover, several new software products were developed in the frame of the project.

From 2005 to 2007 the student was responsible for the design and development of the PACS system in the O3 Consortium project, which has been called O3-DPACS, and for creating and validating the support model on that critical product.

In this thesis the reasons, methods and results of this three years work are described, separated in the following chapters:

Chapter 1 describes the state of the art. It is presented from two points of view: the first concerns the previous experience of the group in *e-health* and clinical data integration, to understand the state from which the student started its contribution to the project, the second concerns the biomedical images management systems, to understand the scenario in which the solutions for O3-DPACS were proposed.

Chapter 2 presents the O3 Consortium project and the several related aspects. In particular, since the student contributed in the team work that led to the definition of the development guidelines, the development model and the business model, these topics will be especially highlighted.

Chapter 3 reports the design of the assistance model realized by the PhD student.

Chapter 4 presents the original solutions chosen by the PhD student to comply and go beyond the development guidelines of O3 project, focusing on the original aspects and research results obtained in this effort.

1

State of the art of healthcare informative systems

1.1: *Concepts and implementations*

The interest in research in biomedical data and signal integration is the principal characteristic of Bioengineering and ICT group of Department of Electrics, Electronics and Informatics of the University of Trieste since early 90s. The highlights of this experience were published in [1].

1.1.1: *The DPACS project*

As a matter of fact, Prof. Paolo Inchingolo led the installation and experimentation of a commercial PACS, a CommView AT&T Philips multi-site PACS system, in 1988 at the Trieste's Hospitals Cattinara and Maggiore. This was also the first installation in Europe of two PACS systems connected together over a metropolitan area network. Despite being this system so innovative for that time and the very positive results obtained with the re-organization of the Radiology Department work, it was early clear that the proprietary installation was forcing users to adapt to the system and not vice-versa. Some issues became evident:

- high running costs
- unaffordable cost of upgrade
- difficulty in creating large archives
- low performance
- no possibility to integrate non-CommView PACS systems and to let them share data
- forced use of expensive customized workstations for data visualization and no easy access from outside the hospitals.

The group work aimed to overcome these limitations of the CommView PACS System and to open the proprietary installation by developing versatile and open source tools (essentially gateways and client workstations) for LAN, MAN and WAN communications with the PACS[2]. By this way, it has been possible distributing

---

[1] Inchingolo P, Beltrame M, Bosazzi P, Cicuta D, Faustini G, Mininel S, Poli A, Vatta F, O3-DPACS Open-Source Image-Data Manager/Archiver and HDW2 Image-Data Display: An IHE-compliant project pushing the e-health integration in the world (2006), Computerized Medical Imaging and Graphics, 30(6-7):391-406

[2] M. Diminich, P. Inchingolo, F. Magliacca and N. Martinolli, Versatile and open tools for LAN, MAN and WAN communications with PACS. In: K.D. Held, C.A. Brebbia, R.D. Ciskowski and H. Power, Editors, *Computational biomedicine*, Computational Mechanics Publications, Southampton (1993), pp. 309–316

images over the hospital departments and surgery rooms of the three hospitals and the bioengineering and medical physics research centers of Trieste, with some connections overseas to the National Institutes of Health at Bethesda, MD (USA), stimulating also the growth of the Informative Trieste System[3]. In 1994, the first PACS browsing interface was developed, allowing virtually world-wide images distribution without dedicated client software[4].

However, as the research, the related results and the clinical experimentation proceeded, it became clear that an impassable limit was reached, due to the intrinsic limitations of the Commview PACS System. For this reason, in 1995 the project of a totally new system named DPACS (Data and Picture Archiving and Communication System) started[5][6].

The goal of DPACS was *"the development of an open, scalable, cheap and universal system with accompanying tools, to store, exchange and retrieve all health information of each citizen at hospital, metropolitan, regional, national and European levels, thus offering an integrated virtual health card of the European Citizens"*.

A first version of DPACS was experimented in 1996–1997 at the Cattinara Hospital[7]. In 1998 the DPACS system was running routinely for managing all radiological images (CT, MRI, DR, US, etc.) as well as in the connection with the stereo-tactic neurosurgery, thus substituting completely the old AT&T Commview PACS system. Some mono-dimensional signals such as ECGs were also integrated into the system. This was the philosophy[8] of this version of the DPACS project.

---

[3] P. Inchingolo, From the GNBTS-NET to the biomedical communication network of Trieste. In: M. Bracale and F. Denoth, Editors, *Proceedings of the MEDICON '92*, Area di Ricerca, CNR, Pisa (1992), pp. 1239–1242.
[4] M. Diminich, P. Inchingolo, N. Martinolli, L. Dalla Palma, P. Giribona and R. Pozzi *et al.*, ARIS: an autonomous remote image station offering both local and remote IMACS/RIS resources in an open environment, *Proceedings of the Third European Conference on Engineering Medicine* (1995), p. 241
[5] F. Fioravanti, P. Inchingolo, G. Valenzin, L. Dalla Palma and R. Vallon, The DPACS Project at the University of Trieste: architecture and working environment, *Proceedeedings of the 14th International EuroPACS Meeeting* Creta, Greece (1996).
[6] F. Fioravanti, P. Inchingolo, G. Valenzin, L. Dalla Palma and R. Vallon, HIS-RIS-PACS integration with the DPACS Project at the University of Trieste, *Proceedings of the 14th International EuroPACS Meeeting* Creta, Greece (1996).
[7] F. Fioravanti, P. Inchingolo, G. Valenzin and P.L. Dalla, The DPACS Project at the University of Trieste, *Med Informat* **22** (1997) (4), pp. 301–314
[8] P. Inchingolo, Trieste and Region Friuli-Venezia Giulia: an example of fully-managed health telematics system the new Telematic Network of 2000's Trieste, *IFMBE Proceedings* **1** (2001), pp. 78–81.

Acquisition Modalities

(TC, MRI, RD, ..)

DPACS server system

Services

Server
DICOM

DICOM

DICOM

HTTP

Gateway

FTP

SQL-NET

Archives
(WORM, DLT)   Local disks   DB Oracle

DPACS workstation

1. **The philosophy of the DPACS project, Version 1997, installed and running routinely at the Cattinara hospital from 1998 to mid 2005.**

Over the years, DPACS was enriched with the sections of anatomo-pathology, anesthesia and reanimation, clinical chemistry laboratory and others; furthermore, its application has been progressively forwarded to the new emerging necessities of the future health care and assistance to the world citizen, based on telemedicine-driven home-care, personal-care and ambient assisted living. The implementation lasted for production from DPACS 97 to 2004 in the hospital of Cattinara in Trieste.

1.1.2: EuroPACS 2004: defining the key points for the problem

In 2004 the group in Trieste organized a huge conference: EUROPACS-MIR 2004[9].

The group, following its project and facing the presented limitations, was working on a new version of the DPACS which was meant to be the next step of the project, retaining all the previous version good solutions, but taking advantage of the acquired experience and the considerations about the new needs, which concerned not only the Cattinara Hospital,

This means mainly the possibility to scale the system easily, according to specific needs and available resources, and the employment of better administration tools to provide a better flexibility to the whole system. Another issue in Cattinara

---

[9] Europacs 2004, www.tbs.ts.it/europacs2004

7

was the integration among different proprietary solutions, to improve the system's capability of interoperating within different contexts, the guidelines suggested by the IHE initiative[10], although not rigidly applied, were implemented. Through modularization and customization, the system was designed to work also in environments that are not IHE compliant, at worst with just slight modifications in code.

The conference brought the major experts of informatics in radiology and healthcare informative system to Trieste. Comparing the DPACS project philosophy to the other experiences all around the world made it clear that several problems encountered during the work in Cattinara where shared among the researchers. Several needs were underlined and they are summarized in picture 2.

The circle of requirements

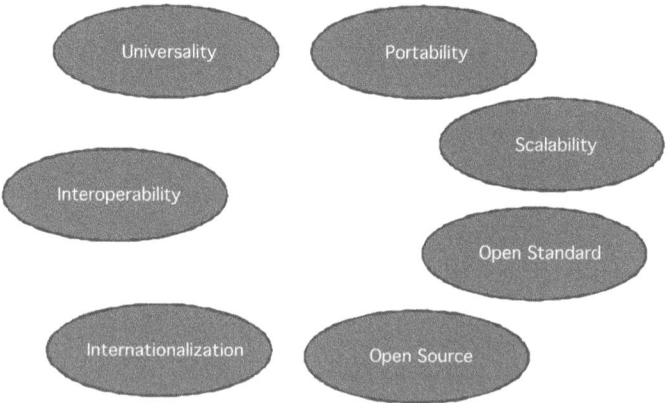

2. The requirements in DPACS project in 2004

The needs were transformed in requirements and it was stated that a state-of-the-art informative system for healthcare should face all the requirements. They were a collection of both DPACS project and euroPACS 2004 outcomes and represent the key point to solve for a successful implementation of technology in *e-health*. They will be explained one by one in the last paragraph of this chapter.

---

[10] Integrating the Healthcare Enterprise web site, www.ihe.net

1.1.3: Premises for O3 Consortium project

In the frame of euroPACS, it was clear that there was a fully compatible project with DPACS one: the MARIS project from Medical and Diagnostic Science and Special Therapies from University of Padua.

After a first experience with the project Raynux (1998), the Department of Medical and Diagnostic Sciences and Special Therapies at the University of Padova developed, starting from 2002, the project MARiS[11], consisting in open tools for the management of the administrative data in a hospital, in particular related to the radiology activity (RIS); in the last two years this work has been extended to the exchange of clinical documents within and among the healthcare enterprises.

The two groups shared the same point of view in using the profiles from IHE initiative and in using only open standards in the development of its products and proposing an open source model. So the O3 Consortium project started, joining the efforts of the two groups. A suite of products was thought, MARIS project bringing its expertise in RIS systems, DPACS project in PACS systems, thus at first a radiology workstation was developed. In particular, in 2004 it became clear that new technologies (JAVA), the growth in maturity of the standards (DICOM, HL7) and the establishment of the new international guidelines for interoperability made the DPACS implementation obsolete and made the group of Trieste think about a new implementation that could, empowering the new instruments, go beyond the accomplishment of DPACS project on its goals.

In 2005 the groups worked together on creating and tuning O3 suite of products. In late 2006 they split because of different points of view on running a business for supporting the project and foster the research. The groups still cooperate on research and development activities.

The PhD student contributed in writing the O3 Consortium project in the three years 2005-2007, with some collaborative work (business model, development model) and some personal original work (such as O3-DPACS design and O3 support model) and led the the validation of the models in the real world.

There is another important premise for O3 Consortium project birth, which is the presence in Trieste of the first European school in clinical Engineering.

---

[11] MARIS project home: http://maris.homelinux.org

1.1.3.1: SSIC-HECE (Scuola Superiore di Ingegneria Clinica – Higher Education in Clinical Engineering)

The interest and the need for some international curricular programs for clinical engineers has been clearly shown since the late 80s by many European transition Countries, as well as by Italy itself to prepare clinical engineering specialists able to implement and work on integrated health systems in the new, enlarging Europe.

The reform of the university studies in Italy and in Europe, according to the Bologna Declaration, has stimulated the transformation of the Specialization School of Clinical Engineering in a new set of curricula called "Higher Education in Clinical Engineering" (HECE)[12]. HECE[13] is spreading the clinical engineering culture in Europe since 1992 and thus the competencies in the evaluation on information technology.

It opened several collaborations among international institutions, hospitals and private companies in order to link all the actors in the clinical engineering market and scientific society. Having so strong connections among users, vendors, law makers and institutions was a great basis to create a living laboratory for the design, development and evaluation of solutions for *e-health* world. O3 Consortium was started also to try to accomplish this aim, in which solutions should be proposed, discussed and contributed by a wide range of actors and an evolving and dynamic sharing of ideas

1.1.3.2: The requirements in the O3 Consortium project

The requirements presented in picture 2 were extended in the frame of O3 project. They are the result of 11 years of research in healthcare systems led by the Bioengineering and ICT group of University of Trieste, the outcome of EuroPACS 2004. They are partially discussed in [14], [15] and build the expanded *"requirements"* circle as stated in the O3 project as follows:

Portability: an healthcare informative system should never force the adopter to any choice in hardware or system software, allowing him to get the most value

---

[12] Inchingolo P, Londero F, Vatta F, The E-HECE e-Learning Experience in BME Education (2007) in: IFMBE Proceedings MEDICON 2007, "11th Mediterranean Conference on Medical and Biological Engineering and Computing", IFMBE Proceedings Series (ISSN:1680-0737), 2007, Ljubljana, Slovenia, CD, pp. 1107-1110

[13] Higher Education in Clinical Engineering website, http://www.ssic.units.it

[14] Fioravanti F, Inchingolo P, Valenzin G, Dalla Palma L, The DPACS project at the University of Trieste (1997), Med Inform (Lond)., 22(4):301-14.

[15] Inchingolo P, Picture Archiving and Communications Systems in Today's Healthcare (1997), WMA Journal (WMJ)

10

from the knowledge of its internal personnel, to increase the reliability and stability of critical systems.

Interoperability: an healthcare informative system should never force the adopter to choices in other software modules which would interact with it. The adopter would be free to choose the best combination of software for his needs and to evolve the system part by part.

Standards: an healthcare informative system should use only open standards, to avoid information being hidden or lost in unknown protocol structures.

Open source approach: having access to the source code and to any change in it, would grant the adopter greater control on the system and more possibilities to survive to failures in the support.

Scalability: an healthcare informative system should implement solutions that could be applied to low load environments up to multicenter systems and regional integration environments. This should foster vertical integration and reduce costs.

Economicity: an healthcare informative system should not force to high investments if not necessary and should try to guarantee the greater reliability at the lowest cost.

Universality: methods and solutions for the healthcare informative system should be exportable to other environments.

These are called design guidelines or requirements. Obviously, these requirements are no-sense if the software lacks in **production level stability, robustness and reliability**.

Moreover, it is still not enough for the healthcare environment because **high level support** is the key to a good implementation of any technology in the real world scenario.

O3 project addresses all these issues and gives a comprehensive answer to them. The validation of the choices has been conducted by the PhD student delivering one of the most critical components in an healthcare informative system: the picture and archiving communication system (PACS), called O3-DPACS. So, finally, the O3 team is proposing a solution for the organization, implementation and managing of a critical informative system in healthcare satisfying all the requirements illustrated in fig.3 and each analyzed deeply through the thesis. The PhD student participated in designing the model, and was in charge of defining the support model, designing the PACS system and performing the validation of the model.

11

The circle of O3 requirements

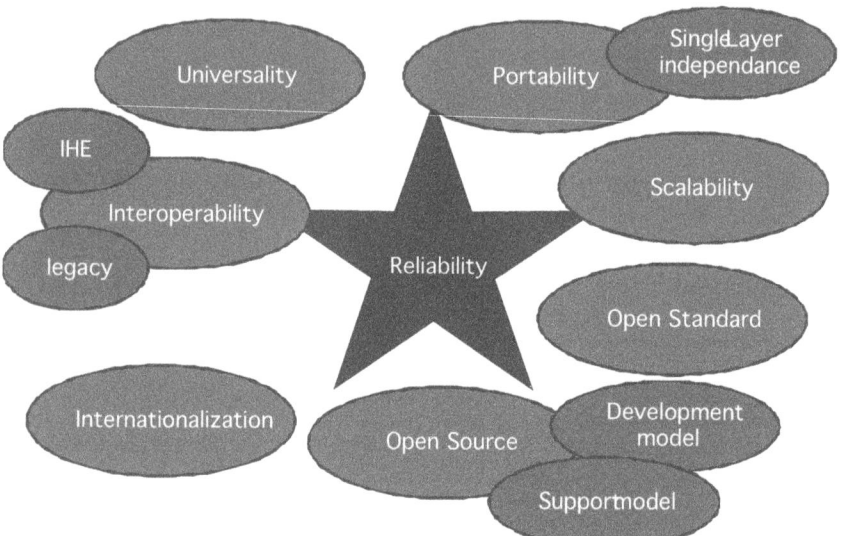

3. **The requirements in O3 Consortium project**

1.1.4: PhD student's role in the creation of O3 Consortium

So, the PhD student's contribution to O3 Consortium was:

- to give a contribution to O3 Consortium project in its foundations, designing a winning model for supporting open source for critical systems, and contributing to the team work for the design of the development and business model.

- to apply and validate the assumptions and the proposed solutions in the sector of PACS systems, because they are the most critical and expensive systems in the actual *e-health* scenario

- to push O3-DPACS to be the best system satisfying the requirements of O3 Consortium project in the market and in the literature, by means of original solutions

1.2: State of the art of PACS systems

The assumptions defined in previous chapter were implemented from 2005 to 2007 in a series of products, called "O3 Suite", meant to be the best *e-health* software according to the *requirements*. The first product design produced on the new O3 requirements was O3-DPACS. Even if the PhD student contributed to the whole work, he personally focused on improving DPACS2004 version to O3-DPACS version of the image manager and archive from 2005 to 2007.

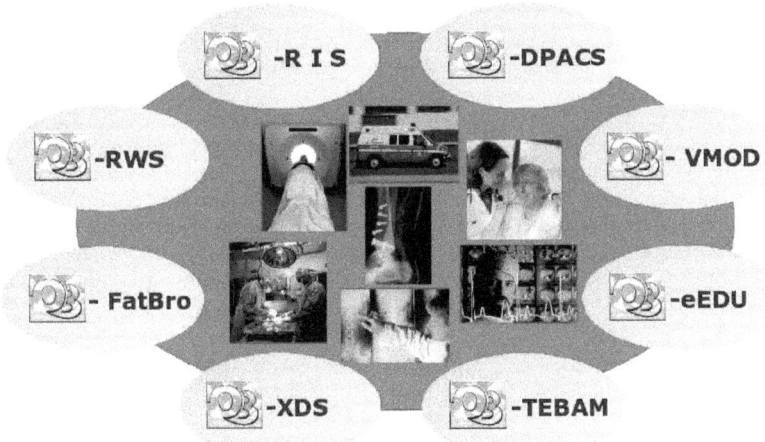

4. The O3 Suite

Besides O3-DPACS, here is a brief description of O3 Suite:

- O3-RWS: O3-Radiology WorkStation is the only Java based radiology workstation running on Windows, Linux and Mac in the world. Taking advantage of long history in biomedical imaging management and manipulation of the Bioengineering & ICT group of University of Trieste the O3-RWS project was started in 2004 and is today on the market. All the assumptions of O3 Consortium project are brought together in the workstation, jointly with one full year of interface research and development in three major hospitals, like Pisa, Padua and Trieste.

- O3-VMOD: O3 Virtual Modality is a simulator of a DICOM modality, the O3 developers team felt there is a lack in the DICOM scenario for a tool allowing you to send, at every time, a new image taken from a predefined set and linking them to a patient taken from a worklist. O3-VMOD was arranged to be used i when instrumentation is not available, for demos, tests or simply didactic purposes

- O3-TEBAM: It allows 3D reconstruction of brain electrical activity from magnetic resonance measurements (MRI) and brain activity mapping even in pathological patients. Today TEBAM researches involve also cluster technologies and high throughput parallel computation strategies and use only open source codes.

- O3-eEDU: is a complete solution for e-learning.

- O3-XDS: O3-XDS, IHE cross enterprise document sharing server (registry and repository) is a brick for joining together information from all the domain of e-health, the three dimensions of the Health Policies - Hospitals, Territory/RHIOs and Home Care/Ambient Assisting Living (AAL). XDS is a IHE profile and an infrastructure that allows the sharing in a "push" model, where documents and data to be shared are "published" to the system. Then, it allows them to be retrieved whichever their physical locations are. O3-XDS is an implementation of the Registry and Repository Actors, entirely in Java and empowers the last J2EE 5 technologies such as EJB3, J2EE 5 persistence and JAXB. Moreover, although being intrinsically multiplatform following O3 philosophy, its advisable platform is the new Glassfish application server.

- O3-RIS: The radiological information system to order, schedule and track exams.

The first product of the suite was a PACS system. The reasons were several:
  - The PACS environment was the one the group had the most experience in
  - Today the PACS system is the healthcare informative system which has the highest cost
  - The system criticism is the highest, as it can be the first level diagnostic engine
  - It's a critical system with high request of support, therefore is the ideal system to test a development and assistance model

Thus, the software was used to experiment the implementation of all the assumption.

Research and technology increase year by year and the current (late 2007) scenario is different from the one from which the studentl started his work (2005). Anyway, the next paragraph will focus on presenting the state of the art from 2004 to 2007 to highlight how the O3 choices and my work fit into it. In the next chapter, how the *"requirements"* turned into implementative, organizational and logistical choices is described.

1.2.1: Literature and market

The literature about archiving and communication systems in medicine has been reviewed and six imaging frameworks projects, plus several commercial products and an open source project have been examined under the light of the *requirements*.

Image archives / managers		Portability DBMS AS OS	IHEIntegrability	Use of standards	Storage format	OS	Scalibility
OpenPacs	2005	Yes / no / no	No	DICOM Jpeg	?	Yes	YES (J2EE, cluster)
Medical Image Data Archive System (MIDAS)	2005	No (C++) / No / No	No	DICOM JPEG web based	?	Yes	Some
Cardiology Solution	2003	No (C++) / no / no	No	DICOM	?	Yes	No
DicomWorks	2007	No (Windows) / No / no	No	E-mail, FTP, or DICOM	?	Yes	No
MyFreePACS	2004	No (C++/php) / no	No	Web	?	?	Some
DICOM Wiki	2005	No(C++/Php) / Postgres	No	Web	?	?	Some
Dcm4chee	2006	Yes / No (Jboss) / Yes	Yes	DICOM Jpeg HL7	DICOM	?	Yes (J2EE)
EyePACS	2004	No (c++, ASP) / No - SqlServer	No	DICOM	On DB	?	No
Medium Comm PACS (2007)	2007	No -Windows / No -Oracle/Sql Server	Yes	DICOM/Jpeg /HL7	Propriet aty	No	No, several products
DPACS	1998	No - C++	No	DICOM	DICOM	No	No
DPACS 2004	2004	Yes / Np / Yes	Yes – SWF	DICOM, HL7	DICOM	No	YES (J2EE)
O3-DPACS	2005	Yes / Yes / Yes	Yes Connectat hon 2006, 2005	Dicom/HL7 Jpeg, Svg	DICOM	Yes Doubl e licens e	YES (J2EE)

The "?" means the information was not retrievable. The "medium commercial PACS" sentence means data have been collected partially by experience and the most from surveys and research from major journals such as *imaging management[16]*.

Reviewing literature, OpenSourcePACS[17], the first reference, is the most complete work available in the contemporary literature about PACS systems. It's a Java enterprise based system building a framework for ordering, processing, reporting and integrating images in the hospital workflow. In the paper, many analogies to O3-DPACS are evident: beyond the technical choices, the open source approach is discussed and the service (assistance) issue for real-world implementation is underlined. In this thesis, the latter will be addressed and the question about if the university environment would suit giving critical services to customers will be answered. Other than OpenSourcePACS, and like O3-DPACS, only DCM4CHEE from dcm4che project[18] is focused on realizing production level PACS systems: it supports IHE, it's Java Enterprise based and community driven. It's the most similar system to O3-DPACS for features. Differences will be underlined in next paragraphs.. The web PACS strategy is deeply analyzed in [19], focusing on the use of WADO service for sharing images over web. We consider it a necessary tool to be used when data load is moderate, while ordinary DICOM and client/server architecture is still needed for full quality reporting. The introduction of multislice CT in the market is increasing the data load per exam to even 1 Gigabyte, pushing to consider different technologies in function of the quality needed by the viewer. If it's a reporting radiologist DICOM client/server technology should suit best, if you're a physician consulting key images, web access via WADO from a web client should be the right choice. Web approach is considered also in DicomWiki[20] and MyFreePACS[21], for promoting the ease of access to every kind of user, the personal use and the use as a reference for research, meetings, and comparisons from any browser enabled PC. EyePacs[22] project considers it a production approach, but ophthalmology exams are less data consuming than state-of-art radiology ones.

DicomWorks[23], while focusing on teleradiology, leverages the necessity of using

16 Imaging management journal web page, http://www.imagingmanagement.org/

17 A. T. Bui. & Kangarloo, H. (2005), 'openSourcePACS: An extensible infrastructure for medical image management', IEEE TRANSACTIONS ON INFORMATION TECHNOLOGY IN BIOMEDICINE, TITB-00168-2005.R1.

18 DCM4CHE project, www.dcm4che.org

19 Norio Nakata, Yasushi Fukuda, Kunihiko Fukuda and Naoki Suzuki, DICOM Wiki: Web-based collaboration and knowledge database system for radiologists, International Congress Series, Volume 1281, CARS 2005: Computer Assisted Radiology and Surgery, May 2005, Pages 980-985.

20 Norio Nakata, Yasushi Fukuda, Kunihiko Fukuda and Naoki Suzuki, DICOM Wiki: Web-based collaboration and knowledge database system for radiologists, International Congress Series, Volume 1281, CARS 2005: Computer Assisted Radiology and Surgery, May 2005, Pages 980-985

21 de Regt, David, Weinberger, Ed, MyFreePACS: A Free Web-Based Radiology Image Storage and Viewing Tool Am. J. Roentgenol. 2004 183: 535-537

22 Cuadros J, Sim I. EyePACS: an open source clinical communication system for eye care. Medinfo 2004;11:207-11

23Puech PA, Boussel L, Belfkih S, Lemaitre L, Douek P, Beuscart R., DicomWorks: software for reviewing DICOM studies and promoting low-cost teleradiology, J Digit Imaging., 2007 Jun;20(2):122-30

DICOM and IHE while the cardiology solution proposed in [24] underlines the need for cost-effective, integrated and open source solutions.

If the literature seems to move to open source approach, with several products available, commercial PACS generally lack an open source approach to protect company investments and know-how. Moreover, they lack scalability, as several products are available on catalogue for the same functions, they lack portability, since compiled languages are generally used for extreme performance and sometimes lack open standards as well, since proprietary solutions are again preferred to optimize performance.

As is shown in the comparison table, O3-DPACS system project today complies as best to all O3 project requirements, that are being generally recognized in the literature as well. The student role was to implement in O3-DPACS the whole set of requirements, and to propose solutions to achieve that goal. For example, an unique step conducted towards the best satisfaction of the requirement is the increase of portability, realized with an original design for O3-DPACS architecture that will be deeply analyzed in the next chapter.

Making a step behind, one crucial point in the effort of complying to all the requirements was the initial platform for O3-DPACS: DPACS2004. The PhD student transformed DPACS2004 in O3-DPACS, and a description of the starting point is needed to understand the improvements.

1.2.2: Dpacs2004

DPACS2004[25] was presented at EUROPACS 2004 in Trieste. DPACS2004 was the version of the PACS system from Bioengineering and ICT group from which the design of O3-DPACS started. Several characteristics where yet implemented and several already named aspects where put under the light.

First, the open source approach: different healthcare enterprises in different countries show several needs and different facilities. DPACS2004 was thought open-source. This policy has been chosen to provide the flexibility needed to promote the adoption of ICT solutions in the healthcare sector in such a heterogeneous environment. DPACS 2004 prototype was thought already to rely on open source software stack. PostgreSQL DBMS running on Linux to store the metadata the application manages was chosen. This seemed a stable solution, efficient for heavy loads and providing features that are not present in other known open-source DBMSs. These include support for different character sets, transactions and concurrent accesses. Experience will then put this in discussion.

---

[24] Marcheschi, P.; Positano, V.; Ferdeghini, E.M.; Mazzarisi, A.; Benassi, A., "An open source based application for integration and sharing of multi-modal cardiac image data in a heterogeneous environment," Computers in Cardiology, 2003 , vol., no., pp. 367-370, 21-24 Sept. 2003

[25] Inchingolo P., Bosazzi P., Cicuta D., Faustini G., Barbaro A., Vittor A. Miniussi E., DPACS-2004 becomes a java-based open-source modular system in proceedings of EUROPACS-MIR, 2004

Open source products were also the libraries to deal with the DICOM standard. The DCM4CHE libraries were chosen, since they are well established, provide an interface to HL7 features as well and are written in Java, the platform that was chosen to implement the application.

As a matter of fact, the proposed solution should be independent in any way of one particular operating system. The almost obvious choice was to use the Java platform. Java was evaluated a robust object-oriented language. As long as a platform is implemented for a particular operating system, a Java application can be run without bothering about native details. Another advantage of the Java platform is that it has been designed to prevent common bugs, mainly in memory management, which can occur often when using other languages. Anyway, operating system independency was not the only requirement, the aim was to be independent from any layer in the needed software stack.

The choice was to use the Java 2 Enterprise Edition to benefit by some additional services it offers. Scalability and messaging are among the most notable, but support for Web services, authentication mechanisms, XML processing or easy access to a DBMS are all features that have been exploited in the project. To actually use these services a normal Java virtual machine is not sufficient. Another application must be installed, a so-called 'application server', which is responsible for providing an implementation of the J2EE platform. The application server is also responsible for providing independency among different DBMSs. This is achieved through a JDBC driver, which implements one of the interfaces in the J2EE platform. As long as one driver is available for connecting to a DBMS, that DBMS can be made available to a Java application. Good application servers exist even as open-source. JBoss 3.0.8 was chosen in 2004, since it was well supported and provided additional features such as clustering.

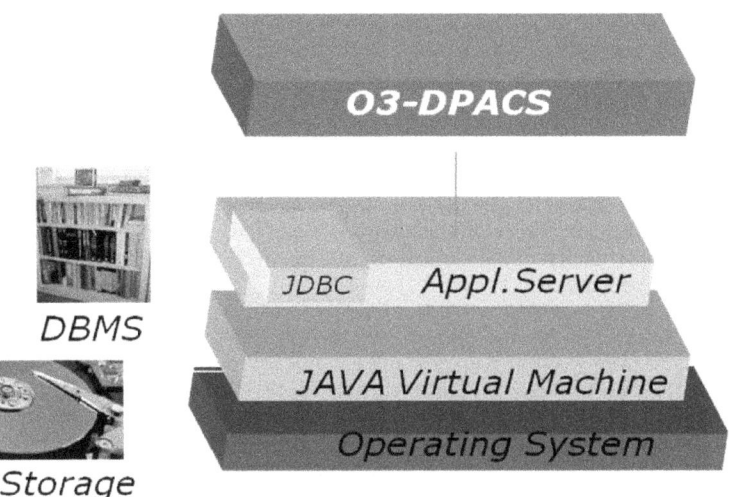

5. The layered stack under O3-DPACS

Clusters represent a set of heterogeneous resources, both hardware and software, interconnected in order to be employed as a single system. This allows an easy management of otherwise cumbersome tasks, as scalability, availability and load balancing. The former is particularly efficient for a DPACS system, since it allows profiting by resource enhancement without restarting the whole application. High availability is crucial to any medical application. A failure in one cluster's element must not compromise the service. In that case clustering allows moving the load to a working element until new resources are added or old ones are recovered.

Another shared aspect with O3 was conformance to IHE guidelines. The proposed solution is therefore meant to facilitate its adoption in several environments, with different hardware and software resources. This doesn't necessarily imply that any platform-independent solution works properly when used in any environment. Experience has proved that many proprietary solutions exist, which cannot interoperate easily. It has been chosen to follow the guidelines suggested by IHE because they are already implemented worldwide, not just in one continent, and because the DPACS project goal is to foster integration among several different healthcare enterprises. This agrees with the choice made in 1995 to use established standards, such as DICOM and HL7. Indeed DICOM and HL7 are the standards suggested by IHE, which is not a standard itself, as some vendors claim, rather a technical framework. It defines entities that participate in some parts of the workflow of an enterprise. The entities are called 'actors' and the parts of the workflow are called 'profiles'. Therefore a system takes part in a profile as some actor.

19

The profiles identified by IHE cover a wide range of common use cases in a healthcare enterprise, from basic scheduling management to charge posting. Suggested actors range from the ADT (Admission/Dismission/transfer) to the acquisition modality. The chosen profiles were SWF, PIR, SEC, known as Scheduled Workflow, Patient Identity Reconciliation and Basic Security.

The enterprises that are, at least to some extent, already IHE compliant definitely don't represent the majority of the existing ones. Some small institutions could not even afford establishing an ICT infrastructure solely to claim conformance to IHE guidelines. This is the reason why we have considered since the start the possibility not to preclude adoption of the new DPACS even in other kinds of healthcare enterprises.

Of course there is no way to make an application integrate immediately in every environment. What was envisioned was an extremely versatile solution, which could integrate to a good extent within many existing health-care environments. Requirements vary sensibly: some may seem odd in rich environments, but may be highly efficient in ordinary enterprises. This can be the case of prefetching or compression. There is no need to prefetch old data, nor to compress them, when you can afford fast lines, but this is not always the case. An enterprise could choose to buy more powerful computers before spending money to enhance the lines. In this case they would benefit by compression facilities and maybe even by prefetching old data during the night. This is the reason why we considered several facilities, organized in switchable modules. This can represent a great benefit for not so rich enterprises and do no harm to rich ones, since they only need to switch the modules off not to waste resources.

Among the main modules, there were the ones for autorouting, prefetching, compression and modality worklists, but every feature of the solution has been designed as a module in order to facilitate management and future expansions. IHE actors, which need to be switchable within an enterprise, are better implemented as module as well, as is the case of the MPPS manager (Modality Performed Procedure Step Manager).

All modules, together with all the system settings, are meant to be managed via Web interfaces. This aspect has been carefully designed, since the former DPACS system lacked administration tools. Settings had to be manually changed, thus requiring specific technical skills from the technician. We believe an IT specialist with knowledge from operating system administration to DBMS management and from application server configuration to software programming is definitely not affordable by ordinary enterprises, such as those which could benefit from prefetching and compression. Access to these interfaces through the Web poses security issues. Not everyone has the rights to modify the settings: this has been simply solved by the obvious employment of AAA (Access, Authentication & Authorization) features and by allowing access only within a restricted network.

Another feature of DPACS-2004 is the presence of several integrated disaster recovery procedures. This concerns the capability to restore the whole system to a consistent state after the occurrence of a failure, a shut-down or a crash. This problem has been solved by employing regular time interval backup functions of configuration files and database tables, by executing a dvd-copy of the operating system resident hard-disk and by logging every operation at several levels. In order to enhance data security, we consider a hardware solution, such as the use of RAID 5 systems.

So DPACS 2004 integrated several choices: IHE, J2EE, open source. From this starting point, two ways should be taken to transform DPACS2004 in a powerful tool that:

- Could be considered for the production application in the real world
- Could be the reference point for data integration and the starting point for healthcare data integration in the citizen life

and finally foster the *e-health* adoption in the world.

One way is developing further the choices made for DPACS2004 moving to the following points:
- Implement the last territorial-level integration profile (leaving the hospital environment)
- Evaluate the reliability of the architecture proposed
- Incorporate new solution to make O3-DPACS remain on the state-of–the–art for PACS systems as in the previous analysis against the *requirements*

The second way is making O3-DPACS an integrated project. This means thinking O3-DPACS as a system that is made of software and of a state-of-the art efficient support model.

The student worked on these two paths while contributing to the creation of O3 Consortium project that fuses the entire discussed topics under a great conceptual umbrella. Should be reminded that O3 Consortium project peculiarity of designing a whole application to real world of open source software in health model is an original effort. No other solution for open source software application makes a complete proposal for all the topics of development, design, software architecture and support. Thus, a real research interest in testing and validating the model can be felt.

2

The contribution to the O3 Consortium project

This chapter describes the reasons and the details of O3 Consortium project. The PhD student contributed in the team work of defining the models presented in this chapter. Moreover, the most relevant methods and materials used for the implementation of O3-DPACS are presented, to allow the reader to understand chapter 4 and 5, where the personal contribution by the PhD student is discussed.

Formally, Prof. Paolo Inchingolo, head of Bioengineering and ICT group in the Department of Electrics, Electronics and Informatics of University of Trieste, started O3 Consortium project in 2005. The project activity was stated as:

to propose a new development model, a new assistance model and innovative software products for healthcare informative systems.

The goal was

to ease the access to technology for every healthcare provider, thus fostering e-health in the world.

The reason for its creation can be found, by the political and organizational point o view as a reaction to two aspects:

1 – The patient is today considered as a passive subject in respect to the healthcare and assistance service provider, instead of being the center of the service

2 – the cost of the healthcare systems is always growing, and the phenomenon will go worse because of the ageing of the world population

From those remarks can be stated that:

The patient concept should be substituted with citizen, who can be ill or health, and healthcare service should mean prevention, assistance and cure, as intended by EU strategies[26].

The citizen should be the center of the organization of the healthcare service, everywhere he would be and everything he's doing.

The Open Three (O3) Consortium project wants to propose a model and some tools to respond to these issues in all the aspects of the citizen ordinary life, summarized in fig.4.

---

[26] Lakovidis, I.; Pattichis, C.S.; Schizas, C.N., "Guest Editorial Special Issue on Emerging Health Telematics Applications in Europe," *Information Technology in Biomedicine, IEEE Transactions on* , vol.2, no.3, pp.110-116, Sep 1998

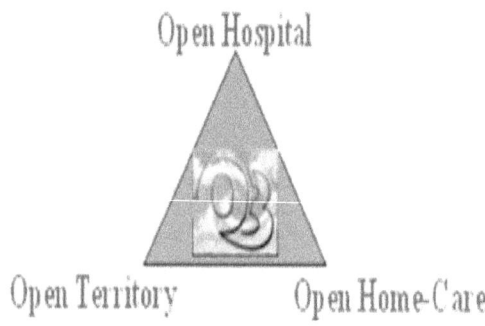

6. The scope of O3 action

The hospital is only one of the environments where the citizen should be supported. The territory, which means preventions and capillary follow-up outside the hospital, should be addressed, and the homecare or mobility care[27], allowing the complete care of citizen health (not disease) should not be discarded.

It is stated in the literature that technology can give a strong help in driving these changes to the health management. Therefore, the spreading of *e-health* adoption can be a factor for a better healthcare service.

As a conclusion, O3 Consortium project was thought as a solution to the whole *e-health* implementation process.
The solution could not be only software or some guidelines, but should consist of single solution for each aspect of a technology implementation:

- Products design guidelines
- A development model
- A support model for products
- A business model for the project auto-sustainability

In this chapter these aspect will be discussed. The support model will be discussed at the end of the chapter, and was created and validated by the writer.

---

[27] Istepanian, R.S.H.; Jovanov, E.; Zhang, Y.T., "Guest Editorial Introduction to the Special Section on M-Health: Beyond Seamless Mobility and Global Wireless Health-Care Connectivity," *Information Technology in Biomedicine, IEEE Transactions on* , vol.8, no.4, pp. 405-414, Dec. 2004

2.1: Design guidelines

The requirements presented in the chapter 1 will be recalled and consequent choices discussed.

Portability: an healthcare informative system should never force the adopter to any choice in hardware or system software, allowing him to get the most value from the knowledge of its internal personnel, to increase the reliability and stability of critical systems.

The portability issue is today solved using Java technology. Literature and market show several examples. The personal experience conducted by the PhD student during the O3-DPACS performance evaluation shows that, accepting a little decay in performances, the technology is mature for critical applications. As a matter of fact, all O3 software modules are written in Java allowing them to be deployed on nearly any operative system. They are all currently tested on Microsoft Windows, Linux and Mac OS/X.

Interoperability: an healthcare informative system should never force the adopter to choices in other software modules which would interact with it. The adopter would be free to choose the best combination of software for his needs and to evolve the system part by part.

In 2000s the initiative "Integrating the Healthcare Enterprise" changed the perspective of the use of open standards. All the O3 products are designed around IHE initiative to best the best interoperable choice as possible. IHE will be presented in the methods section of this chapter.

Standards: an healthcare informative system should use only open standards, to avoid information being hidden or lost in unknown protocol structures.

Only open standard will be used in O3 products. As a matter of fact DICOM, HL7 (Health Level 7), XML , SOAP (Simple Object Access Protocol), HTTP are all open protocols that used in combination can satisfy all the information exchange needs in the healthcare environment.

DICOM, in particular, is spreading its scope of application outside the radiology department and covering signals that were not addressed. The stress test ECG is one of the long awaited data that have been standardized in 2006 version.

Open source approach: having access to the source code and to any change in it, would grant the adopter greater control on the system and more possibilities to survive to failures in the support.

Open source approach needs a separate section to discuss all the implication of its implementation.

Scalability: an healthcare informative system should implement solutions that could be applied to low load environments up to multicenter systems and regional integration environments. This should foster vertical integration and reduce costs.

Scalability is today implemented for servers using Java Enterprise Edition. The Enterprise Edition technology allows one time programming, and the platform is responsible for adapting the code to work load. Moreover, clusters can be done with more machines or services split among machines. This layer allows the programmer to focus on core and architecture, leaving dynamic workload management to the platform. The server components in O3 product suite are all built on J2EE layer. The implementation of the layer is, instead, left to the user with an original solution for portability discusses in chapter 3.

Economicity: an healthcare informative system should not force to high investments if not necessary and should try to guarantee the greater reliability at the lowest cost.

Several of the previous aspects concur to economicity:

- Portability let the user choose the licences of operating systems and database layer he already has, and may be payed for.

- Scalability means lower costs when your workload increases. It's a common situation when informatization is starting.

- Interoperability let the user split the informative system in smaller modules, facing the acquisition of each module separately. This usually leads to optimal contracting and a better product at a lower cost. Then, interoperable products should fit well constituting the complete informative system

- An open source approach means the user can get control of the code if needed and he is less forced to follow the evolution of the serving company

- The use of open standard avoids costs when an integration has to be done or data should be recovered or exported for a failure or simply to share them

Production level stability, robustness and reliability.

It is the first and mandatory requirement for software and of course it is even truer when the software implements a critical system. A critical system is a system requiring high availability and usually is online 7 day on 7 and 24 hours on 24.
In the literature and in the market it is felt a contraposition between:

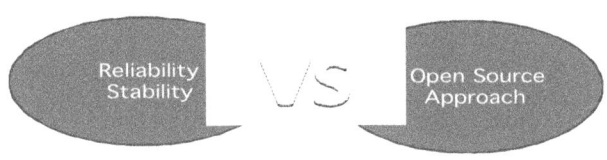

7. Reliability and open source

O3 addresses the problem proposing a development and support model integrated on products that follow the guidelines. So you have that every piece of software is a system with open source approach, with O3 guidelines implemented and a proper development and support model.

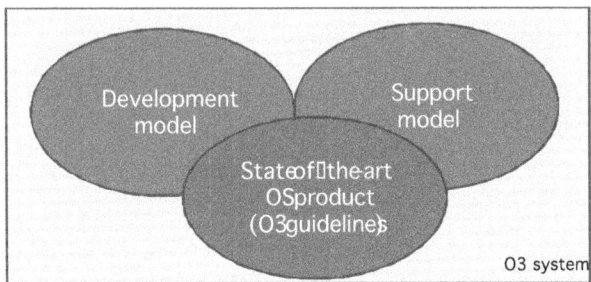

8. The O3 integrated system

Usually the models are the general O3 models but they are sometimes specialized on the products as will be discussed later. The key for the success of the integrated project, besides the quality of the product, is a **high level support.**

Even if the critical system software is of great quality no one would implement it in a critical environment without a specific, quality support.

27

2.2: Methods

2.2.1: Integrating the Healthcare Enterprise initiative (IHE)

IHE initiative is taking a step into market, into tenders and also in the literature; its aims and benefits are widely discussed in [28]. Here is a brief description of IHE useful to understand the topic faced in next chapters.

IHE is an initiative by healthcare professionals and industry to improve the way computer systems in healthcare share information. IHE promotes the coordinated use of established standards such as DICOM and HL7 to address specific clinical need in support of optimal patient care. Systems developed in accordance with IHE communicate with one another better, are easier to implement, and enable care providers to use information more effectively.

More than 100 vendors have implemented and tested products based on IHE. IHE improves patient care by harmonizing healthcare information exchange and provides a common standards-based framework for seamlessly passing health information among care providers, enabling local, regional and national health information networks.

The goals are also:

- Safety through the reduction of medical errors

- Savings through lower implementation costs and more efficient workflow

- Satisfaction through better informed medical decisions and faster results for both patient and physician

IHE follows a defined, coordinated process for standards adoption. These steps repeat annually, promoting steady improvements in integration.

I. Identify Interoperability Problems.

Clinicians and IT experts work to identify common interoperability problems with information access, clinical workflow, administration and the underlying infrastructure.

II. Specify Integration Profiles.

---

[28] Grimes, S.L., "The challenge of integrating the healthcare enterprise," *Engineering in Medicine and Biology Magazine, IEEE* , vol.24, no.2, pp. 122-124, March-April 2005

Experienced healthcare IT professionals identify relevant standards and define how to apply them to address the problems, documenting them in the form of IHE integration profiles.

III. Test Systems at the Connectathon.

Vendors implement IHE integration profiles in their products and test their systems for interoperability at the annual IHE Connectathon. This allows them to assess the maturity of their implementation and resolve issues of interoperability in a supervised testing environment.

IV. Publish Integration Statements.

Vendors publish IHE integration statements to document the IHE integration profiles their products support. Users can reference the IHE integration profiles in requests for proposals, greatly simplifying the systems acquisition process.

Profiles are described in a public document called "IHE Technical Framework".

Each IHE Technical Framework consists of two parts: Profiles and Transactions. IHE Profiles model the business process problem and the solution to the problem; Transactions to support these profiles are defined in detail, using current, established standards to solve the business problem defined by each IHE Profile.

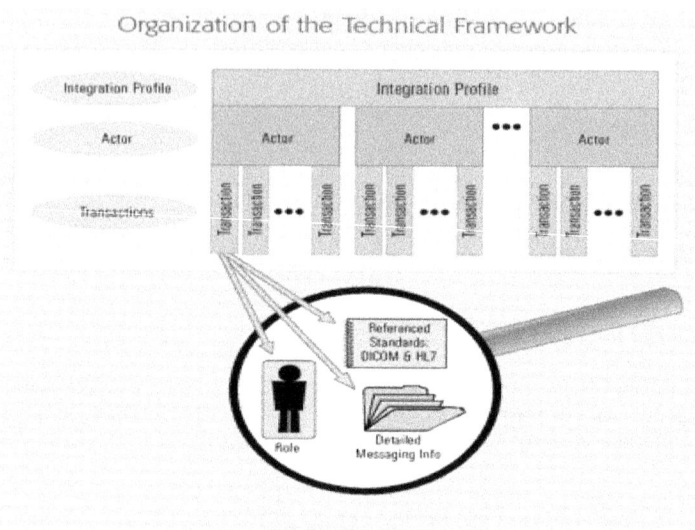

Organization of the Technical Framework

9. **Organization of the Technical Framework**

IHE Profiles are based on the following three modeling concepts: an Actor, a system or part of a system that creates, manages or acts upon data, a transaction. A specific interaction between Actors is needed to exchange information.

IHE Profiles provide a common language for purchasers and vendors to discuss the integration needs of healthcare sites and the integration capabilities of healthcare IT products. They offer developers a clear implementation path for communication standards supported by industry partners and carefully documented, reviewed and tested. They give purchasers a tool that reduces the complexity, cost and anxiety of implementing interoperable systems.

IHE Profiles organize and leverage the integration capabilities that can be achieved by coordinated implementation of communication standards, such as DICOM, HL7, W3C and security standards. They provide precise definitions of how standards can be implemented to meet specific clinical needs. IHE is organized across a growing number of clinical and operational domains such as Radiology, Cardiology, IT etc. Each domain produces its own set of Technical Framework documents, in close coordination with other IHE domains. Committees in each domain review and re-publish these documents annually, often expanding with supplements that define new profiles. Initially each profile is published for public comment. After the comments received are addressed, the revised profile is republished for trial implementation: that is, for use in the IHE implementation testing process. If criteria for successful testing are achieved, the profile is published as final text and incorporated

Each O3 product adheres in some way to IHE, which means it implements a combination of actors and transaction. O3 is discussing profiles into several committees such as PCD (Patient Care Device), is inserted in the technical framework development process and aims to test the new profiles as soon as possible to evaluate their effectiveness. The choice of which profiles to implement and the integration statement will be discussed in next chapters.

2.2.2: Java Enterprise Edition

Java Enterprise Edition raises from the generic need for enterprises to extend their reach, reduce their costs, and lower their response times by providing easy-to-access services to their customers, partners, employees, and suppliers.
Typically, applications that provide these services must combine existing enterprise information systems (EIS) with new business functions that deliver services to a broad range of users. These services need to be

-   Highly available, to meet the needs of today's global business environment.
-   Secure, to protect the privacy of users and the integrity of enterprise data.
-   Reliable and scalable, to insure that business transactions are accurately and promptly processed.

The Java 2 platform, Enterprise Edition (J2EE) reduces the cost and complexity of developing these multi-tier services, resulting in services that can be rapidly deployed and easily enhanced as the enterprise responds to competitive pressures.

J2EE is designed to support applications that implement enterprise services for customers, employees, suppliers, partners, and others who make demands on or contributions to the enterprise. Such applications are inherently complex, potentially accessing data from a multiplicity of sources and distributing applications to a variety of clients.
To better control and manage these applications, their design is multi-tier, to separate presentation, logic and data access layers. The business functions to support these various users are conducted in the middle tier. The middle tier represents an environment that is closely controlled by an enterprise's information technology department. The middle tier is typically run on dedicated server hardware and has access to the full services of the enterprise.
J2EE applications often rely on the EIS-Tier to store the enterprise's business-critical data. This data and the systems that manage it are at the inner-core of the enterprise.

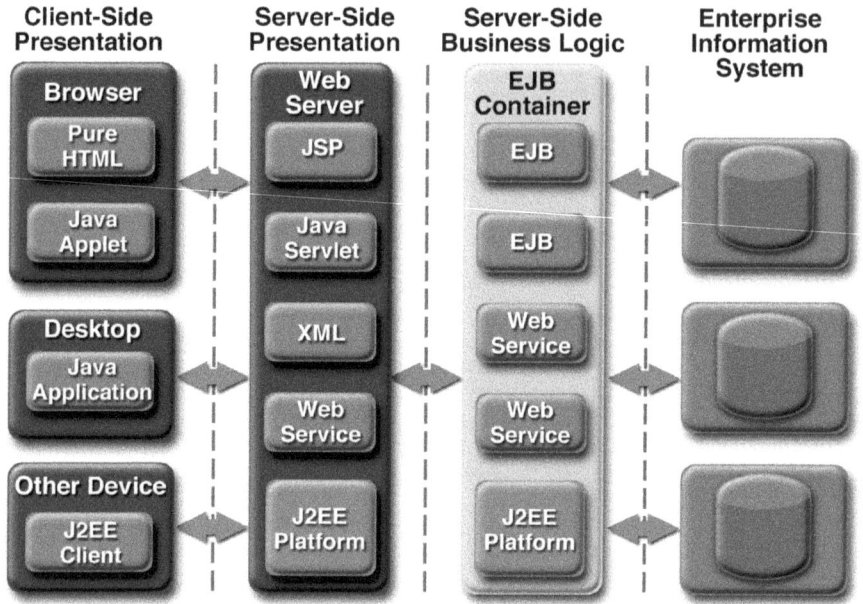

Client-Side Presentation	Server-Side Presentation	Server-Side Business Logic	Enterprise Information System
Browser Pure HTML, Java Applet	**Web Server** JSP, Java Servlet, XML, Web Service	**EJB Container** EJB, EJB, Web Service, Web Service	
Desktop Java Application			
Other Device J2EE Client	J2EE Platform	J2EE Platform	

10. The tiers of Enterprise Application

Multi-tier applications provide the increased accessibility that is now demanded by all elements of an enterprise. Developing multi-tier services has been complicated by the need to develop both the service's business function and the more complex infrastructure code required to access databases and other system resources. Because of each multi-tier server product had its own application model, it was difficult to hire and train an experienced development staff. In addition, as service volume increased it was often necessary to change the whole multi-tier infrastructure, resulting in major porting costs and delays.

The J2EE application model defines architecture for implementing services as multi-tier applications that avoid these problems and deliver the scalability, accessibility, and manageability that is needed.

The J2EE application model partitions the work needed to implement a multi-tier service into two parts: the business and presentation logic to be implemented by the developer, and the standard system services provided by the J2EE platform. The developer can rely on the platform to provide the solutions for the hard system level problems of developing a middle-tier service.

The J2EE application model provides the benefits of *Write Once, Run Anywhere*™ portability and scalability for multi-tier applications. This standard model minimizes the cost of developer training while providing the enterprise with a broad choice of J2EE servers and development tools.

The following standard Java service APIs are an example of J2EE services and are the basis of an enterprise application design:

- JDBC™ - the standard API for accessing relational data from Java.
- Java Naming and Directory Interface™ (JNDI) - the standard API for accessing information in enterprise name and directory services.

They are implemented in O3–DPACS and therefore will be discussed later in the thesis.

Finally, it is important to remark the "container" concept. It's a space where certain types of classes live, like web classes in the web server, and gives services to those classes. When you write an Enterprise Java Bean class (EJB), it must be deployed in a container, the container layer becomes aware of the EJB and can, for example, manage pools of the classes you've written to achieve high availability. This concept and its components are (out of scope for the moment) depicted in the figure.

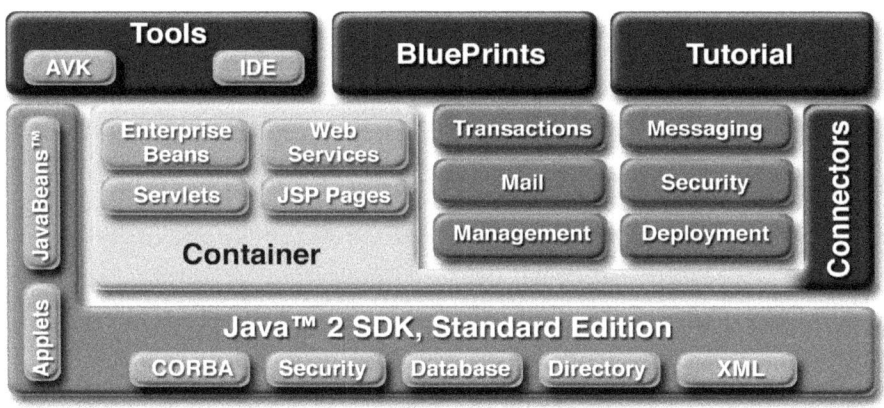

11. The container in the Java EE structure

2.2.3 Java Management eXtensions

Enterprise adoption of J2EE as the strategic architecture for server-based applications is on the rise. Increasingly, mission-critical applications are being built and deployed on J2EE infrastructures. This trend is driving demand for better administration, monitoring and management of J2EE applications as well as the underlying network and systems infrastructure. J2EE based solutions will need to deliver on the management needs of large enterprises to be successful. An emerging standard, Java Management Extensions (JMX), will be essential to meeting these needs for J2EE applications.

While JMX is widely being used for managing J2EE infrastructure, the most interesting aspect of this technology is that it enables powerful management capabilities for the applications themselves. This goes beyond managing just the J2EE server or other middleware infrastructure. This ability to easily and directly manage the specific applications built on J2EE or other infrastructure is a major benefit of this technology.

A promising aspect of JMX technology is the business benefits it promises beyond basic application management. Many mission-critical software deployments support business processes that need to be monitored and mined for information that drives key business decisions. JMX makes it easier to quickly expose information on demand from critical systems used in operating the business, and to use that information for business intelligence and informed decisions. As an example you can monitor the valuable resources of your PACS application, such as DICOM clients connected, memory used, query done, to have a view on your application status and make wiser decisions in case of failure or malfunctioning.

Most application developers view management as an afterthought when building and delivering their applications. In some cases, developers try to anticipate administration and monitoring needs of their users, and build such administration, logging and instrumentation into their applications. This often uses a variety of proprietary mechanisms for consoles, log files, and instrumentation. While this may fulfill the immediate needs anticipated by application developers, it is usually a poor fit with the real requirements of enterprises that have to deal with a complex integration of many such applications. If each application has its own way to do administration and monitoring, handling the diversity of management tools becomes its own challenge.

There is therefore a need for standards-based instrumentation from applications, such that the management applications can use it effectively.

JMX is a Java standard that specifies a model and the interfaces for remote or local management of Java applications. An important goal for JMX is to allow a broad range of management systems and applications access to instrumentation and control of the managed applications. JMX achieves this goal with a creative model that uses a common set of application management components and provides access via multiple protocols like SNMP (....) and HTTP. With JMX, applications can be instrumented once and be managed via multiple protocols accessing the same management instrumentation. Furthermore, it allows for rapid manageability in ways that no longer require heavy lifting by application developers.

The architecture for JMX is illustrated in Figure 12. The goal of enabling remote management from different kinds of management applications and systems is solved with a layered approach.

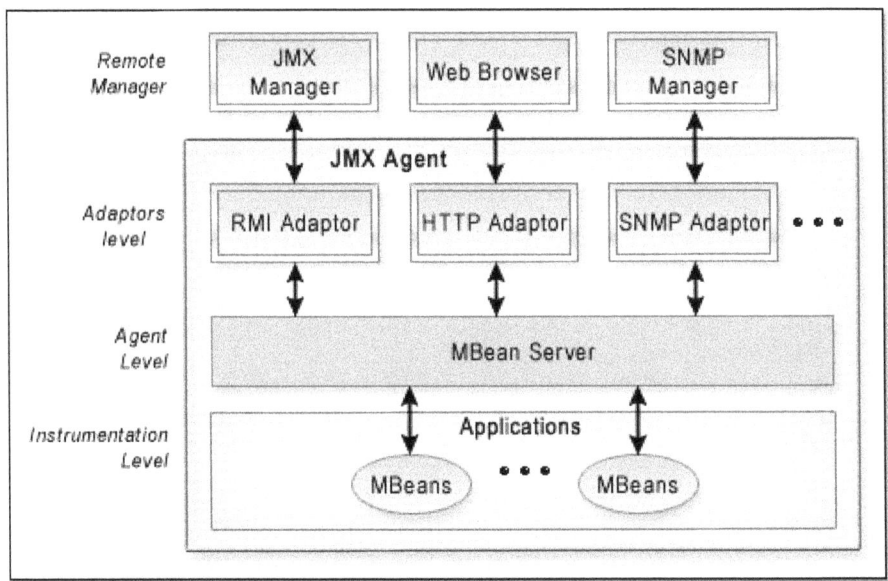

12. The JMX structure

At the application level (called the Instrumentation Level), components called MBeans provide the application-specific management information. These MBean components, which bear some similarity to Java Beans, provide the essential visibility and control for managing applications. These components interact with the applications and are developed for each application based on its management needs. For example, an MBean may provide a method to shutdown an application component.

The Agent Level interfaces the MBean components and provides a management interface to these components. The MBean Server is the key component in this layer, and provides a set of management functions useful to manage MBeans.

The Connector Level, or the Protocol Level, consists of one or more connector (or protocol adaptor) components that provide access to remote management systems.

Depending on the protocols supported by the JMX implementation, remote managers supporting SNMP, HTTP, or other management protocols can access the management information and control exposed by the MBeans for each application. Multiple management systems using different protocols can now simultaneously access the application management capability. Thus the application management can be made available to existing enterprise management consoles traditionally used in enterprises.

The MBean components are Java classes that fit design patterns based on the type of MBean. The defined MBean types are Standard, Dynamic, Open and Model MBeans. Standard MBeans provide a static interface. Dynamic MBeans provide an interface that can change at runtime, and is defined by metadata associated with the MBean. Open MBeans are Dynamic MBeans that use a small set of universal Java types. A Model MBean is a Dynamic MBean that provides a generic template for managed resources, so that users can expose the information they want without creating MBean classes.

JMX includes a complete notification model so MBeans can easily generate notifications, and managers can register for and get asynchronous notifications. These notifications are supported over each of the management protocols integrated with the JMX agents.

A common need for modular application architectures is a component model that can be remotely controlled, including adding, starting and stopping modules. JMX provides a great standard solution for this purpose, and enables applications to take advantage of its modular, extensible, lightweight architecture for this purpose. Some J2EE application servers, e.g. JBoss, use JMX as the core application control infrastructure. With this approach, standard application consoles, including HTML consoles, can be readily provided once JMX is integrated into the infrastructure.

By eliminating protocol and connector dependency cleanly from the MBeans and application instrumentation, JMX makes a number of other benefits possible. Management access to information and control of applications has always depended on providing this access through appropriate instrumentation. Through this simple but rich component model for creating the instrumentation, JMX makes it easier for developers. More importantly, it makes possible automated tools to generate instrumentation and radically simplify the burden on the application developer. This new breed of tool empowers the developer to quickly and easily provide the kind of information needed to properly manage his application.

An important consequence of this kind of tool is the ability to add and change the management information and control being exposed without touching or disrupting the application code itself. As a result, manageability can be added or changed at any time in the product lifecycle. As many application developers know, the management requirements sometimes change when the rubber meets the road. This type of tool allows for meeting these changing requirements, without the long delays associated with any change in the application code.

The PACS application monitors several variables at runtime. A problem was the lack of a standard infrastructure to execute the monitoring and a standard implementation on which rely. DPACS2004 was linked to its lower stack (Application Server with custom JMX implementation) and O3-DPACS taking advantage of this JMX technology made a step beyond towards portability breaking that link. More details are in the next chapter.

2.2.4 The growth of DICOM standard scope

DICOM standard is today covering more than the radiology environment. From 2004 several extension are being considered and continuously updated. Examples are the introduction of ophthalmic SOP classes like Ophthalmic Coherence Tomography (OCT), Storage SOP Class implementing the encapsulation of documents like PDF and DICOM Encapsulation of HL7 reports. Moreover, Radiotherapy (RT) Structure Set, Plan, Dose, Treatment Record, Waveforms (ECG, Hemodynamic, Audio), Enhanced CT Image, Veterinary, X-ray angiography are only a few of the argument in ballot.

Since DICOM is a standard-de-facto, continuously updated and not related to a specialty (radiology) it is the best vector for interoperability.

2.3: *The O3 development model*

The O3 development model, thought by O3 project team with the PhD student contribution, specially related to the release system and considerations on the opportunity of the double license system, consists of:

- a core team (O3)
- a developer community
- a user community and a service provider community.

O3 Consortium university staff and members from O3-Enterprise represent the core team. The core team work together with a medical experts team to drive the development, choose the roadmap and the objectives of the projects. It is responsible for research, for the development of the code, for education on O3 themes. Moreover, jointly with the enterprise members, is responsible for quality evaluation, test and eventually integration of the contributions by external developers.

The core team collects inputs from the user community such as feedbacks on the products, evaluates them and plans the development of O3 suite accordingly. The development model is today integrated with hard tests, and will be regulated with a quality control policy in next months.

O3 core team is also responsible for releasing the software. The PhD student contributed to the decision to use the double license model, putting several reason under the light. Generally, a version is released twice or three times a year as GPL General Public Available license. The software is therefore downloadable *"as is"* from Internet without any guarantee and freely implementable by users. A simple registration is needed to verify developers claimed identity, and to be allowed to download the software. Public CVS (Concurrent versioning system), currently opened on *sourceforge.net*, are a vector for contribution and O3 Team is responsible to monitor them and "promote" them into commercial or GPL version. It has been chosen to deliver different version on the O3 website or *sourceforge*. On the latter, collaborative tools are used and the community version is growing, on the first ready-to-use installation packages are available. More details on this choice will be given in the last chapter.

The drawback of GPL version is the lack of guarantees that a company can give on the code in the terms of bug fixing and code personalization.

The commercial license addresses these needs and is more suitable for healthcare application, where the same open source code, or it plus commercial add-ons are delivered, covered by strict guarantees regarding intervention time, time to solve bugs, time for updates delivering. The commercial code is updated continuously, whereas GPL code is updated on voluntary basis let's say three times a year. It's allowed to community to build its fork or un-validated add-on, O3 will reserve to try it, test and choose wether to include in the original distribution or not.

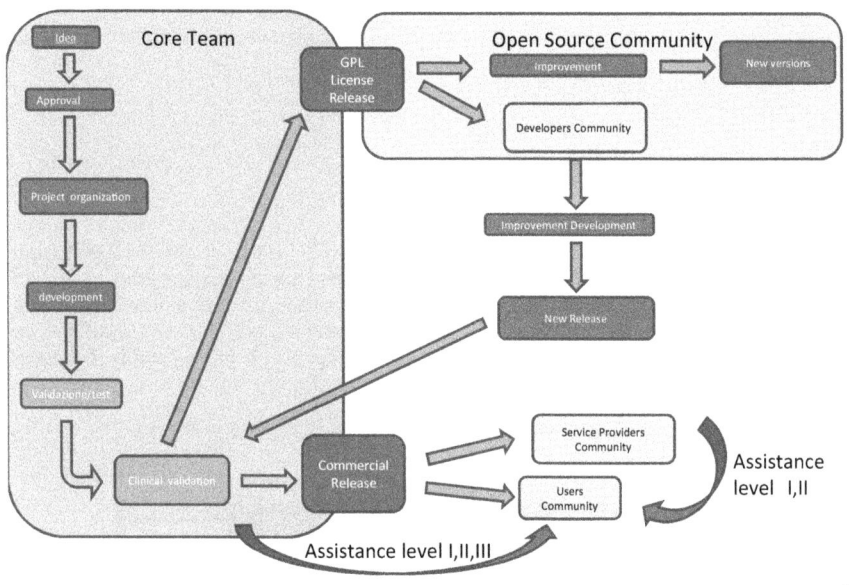

13: Development model

What was even more important, according to the PhD student research, was the importance of the commercial licence in the context of medical application. Commercial license is mandatory to have CE certification, which is needed for medical use for production. In this case the quick evolution of versions of typical open source products is not suitable to be certificated, but a vendor can certificate an open source specific version of the code. O3 Enterprise will do it on specific version, completed by manuals and necessary documentation, to allow professional open source use.

It must be said that a great obstacle to professional opensource in healthcare is the fact that CE certification is deeply linked with quality of production system. As a matter of fact neither a community neither the university can afford the effort of certification and the expence in setting up a quality system. This is a matter that can be overcomed when exist a hi skilled entity which can take care of quality, certification and responsibility of open source medical software.

As a matter of fact, since software from 2007 is a medical device, cannot be used professionally in health care without certification.

An issue is about intellectual property and ownership of the code. The owner of the code is the University of Trieste, in particular prof. Paolo Inchingolo as the leader of the research of Bioengineering and ICT group, and being the person who ideated and decided the direction of the research. The O3-Enterprise and O3 Consortium project staff today can deliver the best license for the release of the software as they have been, and are, co-authors and co-researchers in the frame of the O3 project.

2.3.1: The O3 Consortium web site

O3 Consortium web site (www.o3consortium.eu) is the host for the beginning of any collaborative task among O3 core, developers and user communities. The site was put online in the actual version in august 2007 and counts one new registered contact per day. The site is built on Joomla[29], an open source content manager to build web site. The huge availability of plug-ins for any need, such as user management or file repository is one of the reasons for the choice.

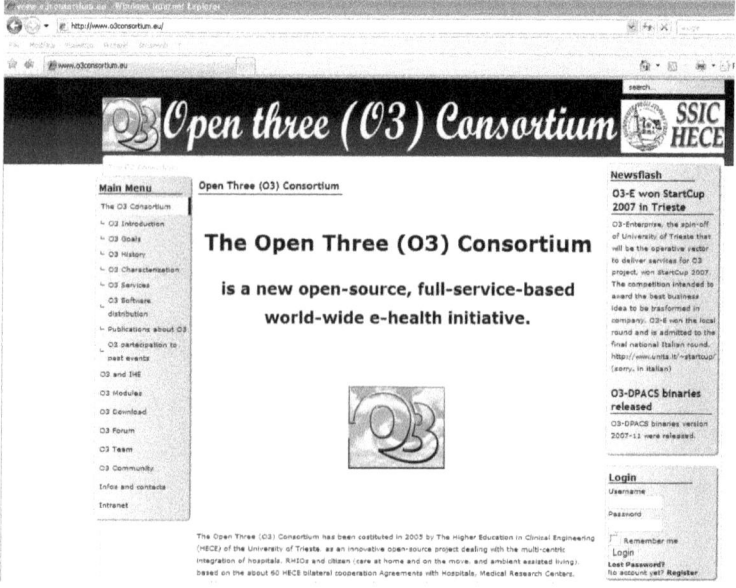

14: O3 Consortium website

_____
[29]Joomla, content manager system, http://www.joomla.org/

Nowadays the most important areas, besides project and modules description, is the download area, where software can be found, and the forum, where discussion about *e-health* topics is encouraged and questions about the installation of the products can be posted.

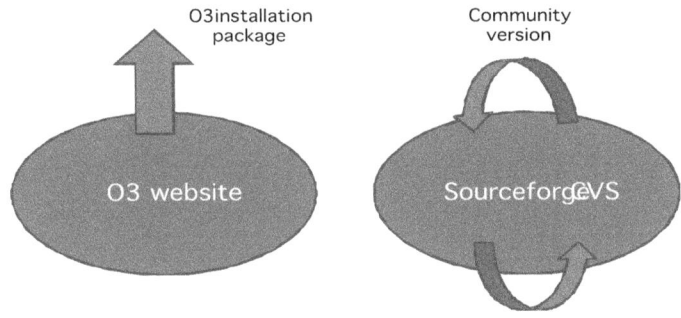

15: O3 code download and collaboration sites

The PhD student chose the source code to be available on *Sourceforge* (www.sourceforge.net). The reasons are worldwide availability, less problems for backup and great visibility. Of course even who is out of *e-health* world would recognize *Sourceforge* as the reference point for serious open source projects. O3 wants to use *Sourceforge* as main platform for the development while using O3 website from a second point of view. Moreover he found that people wanting more information about the software, or wanting a tested and prepared installation package, or information about services, guarantees and offers, would visit the O3 website as the complete guide to satisfy those needs. He also felt that the non-mandatory registration needed to post to the forum and download is not a stress but a sign of good behavior and serious intent. On O3 website are of cource available all the information to obtain a commercial license with support.

2.4: O3 Business Model

While putting together the theoretical model of O3 Consortium, it was clear that also the auto-sustainability of the initiative should be addressed, by an economic point of view.It has been said in the previous chapter that, for many reason concerning support, certication and guarantee, a juridical subject should take of the open source product. To do so, the concept of spin off company called O3-Enterprise was included in the model.

The company should have some specific characteristics to comply to the business model been thought by O3 team. The company should be an university spin-off (in this case of the University of Trieste) and should be the operative part of O3 Consortium project. Since the creation of the enterprise and its sustainability is the result of all the conceptual and practical work on O3 Consortium project, it will be discussed in the last section of the thesis.

Here, a brief description of the ratio for its creation and about where the business is, is described in this section.

Until 2008, the department of the University that was dealing with the administrative task for O3 activity faces some difficulties:

The university cannot move fast in the marketing world
The university have lot of burocracy
The university cannot afford effective contracts for working personnel
A contract that passes through the university is cut by taxes

On the other hand, being a part of a University presents some advantages:

The university is the right place for research and stay on the state-of-art edge
The university cannot die, versus ordinary company
The university can be the right partner to public administration

Anyway, a company can have its own advantages:

Can go directly to customers with efficient marketing
Can deal without constraints with personnel

Although:

A starting company does not have any credibility to go in the healthcare market

So, to take the best from all the aspects, a complex structure has been designed.

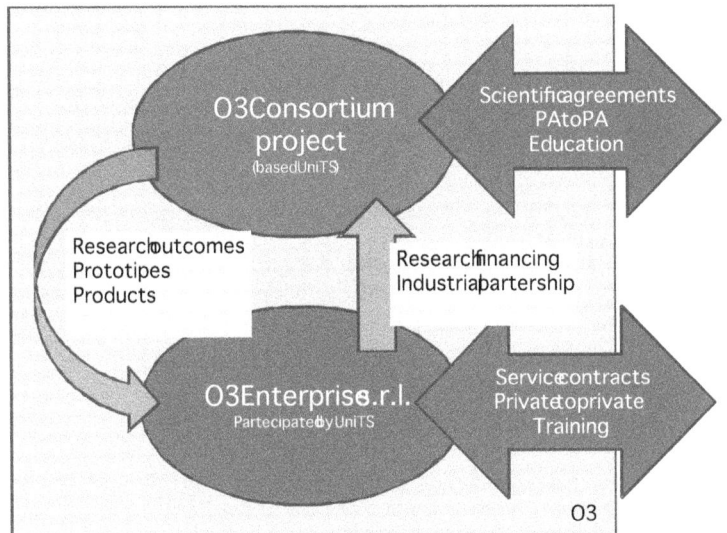

16: O3 Consortium project/Enterprise structure

O3 consortium project should continue to be run at University, and should conduct research, education and initial product prototyping and development. Then an enterprise should be created to deliver services over products and take care of distribution, marketing add engineerization of the products.

Both the entities would have their best interlocutors customer from the public administration area for the University and private healthcare providers, service providers and IT company for the enterprise.

The O3 Consortium project would assign the service and share the knowledge on the products to O3 Enterprise as special partner, which will recognize an amount of money taken from its earnings as a support for O3 research.

This mutual support of the two entities seems to make the structure self-sustainable and capable to join all the best aspects of the two juridical entities.

Another particular issue is the training for service provider option. Since O3 does not aim to grow as a multinational company, but aims to foster technology adoption by adoption of its software modules, the vision is that several institutions or companies should provide first and second level assistance in the world. It means that they can go physically to the customer in case of failure and also solve configuration mistakes or optimize the installation. Third level support, which basically means modifying the code for improvement or correction is always assigned to the O3 core team. Eventually, the bug fixing or the proposed addiction to code can be proposed to the O3 team.

O3 Consortium team provides training for such entities and continuous education to keep knowledge in the systems at top level. This is an original characteristic of O3 development and support model.

At the same time O3 "bricks" are proposed to companies willing to integrate them into their complete systems.

This way for O3 modules development and distribution aims to spread the technology and constitute a modern technological substrate to allow next-day applications and research.

2.4.1: O3 Enterprise

As a consequence of the discussion carried on during this thesis, the company to give professional and commercial services on O3 product suite has been created. The company takes advantage of the scientific collaboration started by O3 Consortium project that are transforming in service agreements or service providing collaborations. Here is an example of the last (2007) roster.

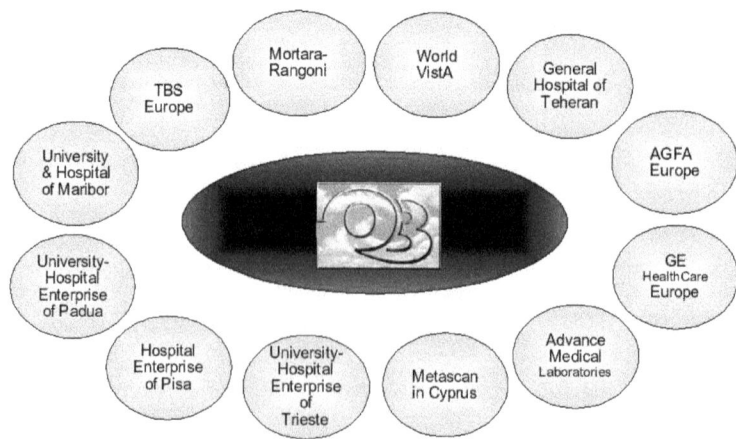

17: The net of O3 collaboration and services in 2007

The company effort is shared among the O3 Consortium staff, the University of Trieste and an industrial partner, ItalTbs S.p.a..

A business plan was written and presented to Start Cup University competition, the competition which award the best idea for a company at the University and won in the year 2007 the edition in Trieste.

The company was juridical started in December 2007 and is now giving services to three installation and developing software in radiology, cardiology and telemedicine for the European market.

3

The definition of the assistance model

The student defined the assistance model for O3 products. His solution is reported in [30] and in the present chapter. As a premise, it should be remarked again that in the real world, the open source approach is spreading, but the *e-health* environment faces some peculiar issues, as described in the previous chapter, and recognized in the literature. The benefits of the approach, in fact, are widely felt. An example is the increase in interoperability and cost effectiveness, which is presented either in [31] and [32]. In the literature, the need for cost-effective, integrated and open source solutions is underlined either in the imaging sector, in projects such as OpenSourcePACS[33], either in the cardiology one[34]. The analysis by McDonald[35] states that today *"the open source approach has gained a tiny foothold in healthcare"*, but there are still hard discussions about some drawbacks. One of them is the difficulty in performing strict quality control for the software produced by open source communities[36], then, the difficulty to gain conformance and certifications for open source healthcare software, in [37] about Osirix and, finally, the need for dedicated support is addressed in the paper describing the OpenSourcePACS project from University of California. In the paper, beyond technical choices and description, the open source approach to healthcare software is discussed, and the service (assistance) issue for real-world implementation is underlined: in particular, the critical aspect of the possibility for an University to deliver support services to customers is discussed.

But to answer the questions and overcome University limits, as it has been told in the business model presentation, a spin-off at the University of Trieste, including some institutional and industrial partners has been created to deliver all the services on O3 software. The University will participate the company, providing a

---

[30] Beltrame M, Ambrogi F, Bosazzi P, Carrara A, Frescura F, Poli A, A new support model for open source critical systems in healthcare: the O3-DPACS experience, accepted to EuroPACS 2008.

[31] Ratib O, Swiernik M, McCoy JM, From PACS to integrated EMR (2003), Computerized Medical Imaging and Graphics, 27(2-3):207-215.

[32] Dinevski D, Inchingolo P, Krajnc I, Kokol P, "Open Source Software in Health Care and Open Three Example" (2007), Computer-Based Medical Systems, 2007. CBMS '07. Twentieth IEEE International Symposium on , pp.33-40, 20-22 June 2007

[33] Bui AT, Kangarloo H., 'openSourcePACS: An extensible infrastructure for medical image management' (2005), IEEE TRANSACTIONS ON INFORMATION TECHNOLOGY IN BIOMEDICINE, TITB-00168-2005.R1.

[34] Marcheschi P, Positano V, Ferdeghini EM, Mazzarisi A, Benassi A, "An open source based application for integration and sharing of multi-modal cardiac image data in a heterogeneous environment" (2003), Computers in Cardiology, 367-370

[35] McDonald CJ, Schadow G, Barnes M, Dexter P, Overhage JM, Mamlin B, McCoy JM, Open Source software in medical informatics--why, how and what, (2003), International Journal of Medical Informatics, 69(2-3):175-184.

[36] Zhao L and Elbaum S, Quality assurance under the open source development model, Journal of Systems and Software, 66(1):65-75.

[37] Ratib O and Rosset A, Open-source software in medical imaging: development of OsiriX (2006), International Journal of Computer Assisted Radiology and Surgery, 1(4):187-196

great guarantee of stability and long-term partnership over ordinary companies.

The double license model, the "moderated" community model and the assistance model used in O3 were chosen to face the need for reliability in the e-health world trying to join it with an open source community model. Since no healthcare provider would use a software "as is" or without proper support, O3 Consortium project was thought as an integrated project, selling commercial state-of-the-art services on open source free products.

Moreover, healthcare providers implementing technology struggle looking for the optimum among the quality of service, economy, growth of internal knowledge in technology applications and security.

The issues to reach the goal are:

- the cost of the resident personnel that a critical system like a PACS needs
- the fact that tenders and investment planning usually include several voices. Those can be more effectively faced separately
- the opportunity of taking advantage of any available knowledge internal to the customer, by example if the healthcare providers owns sufficient competencies in hardware and systems
- the need for fast failure response time should be faced, usually driving to the need for a reliable service structure

Thus, the PhD student created the following assistance model for customer requiring its services. The software is delivered as open source, but with a commercial license that protects the healthcare provider with guarantees on bug fixing, updating, and failure recovering.

Support services are structured in a convenient way. Every installation has two responsible, one from O3 and one from the customer, who usually sign the support contract. Then, an operative team is composed. One person is the one from O3 enterprise?? that knows all about the specific installation: wards, workflow, equipment installed, and is called "*project manager*". The second should be provided by the customer: he is responsible for hardware and systems, meaning operative systems and general applications. A third person playing as interface to the users: physicians and other personnel is also supplied by the customer. This team consolidates all the knowledge needed to take operative decisions, and, more important, to join experience on different levels for problem solving. It could be argued that two resources provided by customer could be a high cost. On the contrary, on one side no one of this team is forced to do exclusively this task, since medium involvement is not full time, on the other side the participation to the team allows the customer personnel to use and develop skills that can be used transversally among applications and different target users. For example, systems management skill can be applied to all installed software to use a single enterprise wide approach, or expertise in starting a service in a ward can be reused in another ward. It should be underlined that these skills should remain internal, in the customer enterprise and can be a factor for the growth for its quality of service.

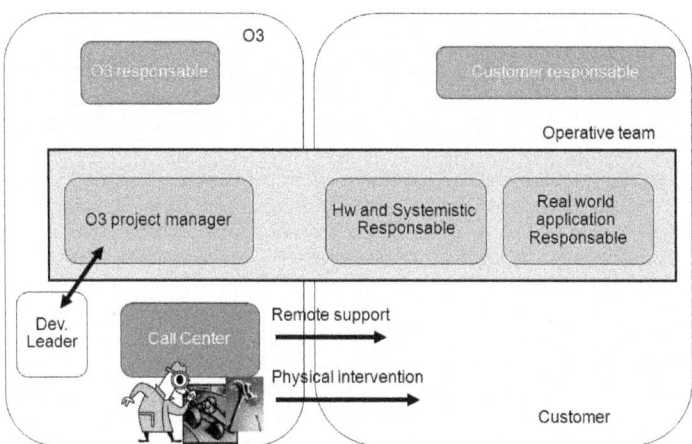

Figure 18: The O3 assistance model

To deliver 7 days on 7 and 24 hours on 24 support service, a call center is provided by O3. It provides toalert the project manager in any case of not urgent tasks, allowing him to decide for the most appropriate action or routes the request for direct intervention by technicians as needed: remotely if possible or onsite when needed. The project manager acts linked to development leader of each supported product, to evaluate if fixing is needed or modification to the development road-map should be considered.

O3 effort is to keep the project manager and technicians as close as possible to the development process, even assigning them a part in it. This should highly increase personnel awareness and knowledge in the product in order to deliver a better support service.

The key point for the sustainability of this model is the use of software technology for remote intervention: SSH tunneling, virtual private networks, terminal access. These are mature technologies and, if well administrated, are the best way to open healthcare networks to external support.

Finally, the proposed support model seems to reach the following goals:

- reduce support costs for O3, and for the customer as a consequence, due to the optimal use of remote support strategy
- reduce the cost for the customer, assigning to the support team only task shared personnel developing useful skills for the enterprise
- increase quality of service, since a team with a great skill in problem solving can be constituted, sharing different competencies either from customer and either from service provider

49

The product supported by the described assistance model was tested in several environments. It is in use for production in environments varying from the departmental installation in Santa Chiara hospital in Pisa, working with good performance on an ordinary pc using an AMD Athlon XP 3000+, 2 GB RAM and a 2 Tb NAS storage, to the Padua hospital installation, where O3-DPACS runs on a virtual machine on professional virtualization hardware, managing 120.000 exams per year and three levels of storage using all modern storage technologies.

Good performances mean that from user perspective a query against current day exams should last less than 5 seconds and the time for retrieving a study should remain in the order of the network transfer time. Obviously, to be referred as good performances, they should remain stable on the long period and do not degrade in significant way.

The validation was conducted, both during 2005 and 2006, at the Azienda Ospedaliera in Padua and at the Azienda Ospedaliero-Universitaria in Pisa. From June 2006, O3-DPACS was in production with regular support contract in Padua, with regular research agreement in Pisa, both using the same support model. The agreements were renewed in June 2007 and all the parties agree that the model is worth the effort made by healthcare providers to use some human resource for it. O3 personnel was forced to only three on site interventions in more than two years for Padua and one for Pisa. One for DBMS migration, two for strategic meetings, another one for a major upgrade and database improvement. Hospital personnel is aware of O3-DPACS features and development roadmap, and therefore understands its strengths and weakness: this allows them to optimally integrate it in the hospital workflow and in any future project, and promptly react to the minimal malfunctioning, providing the best information for the most effective intervention by O3 team.

The live two year working experience with hospitals of Padua and Pisa seems to be the best validation of O3 support model and is the first example in Italy of production open source PACS environment, with external support.

The assistance model was validated in two major Italian hospitals and proved to be reliable in different environments, with different requirements, as described in the result section. The renewed fidelity in the product and in the support, proved by the fact that all experimental installations turned to real service agreements and all are being carried on, testifies that the obstacles to the open source approach adoption can be overcome.

4

The O3-DPACS challenges and original aspects

4.1: O3-DPACS architecture

O3-DPACS expanded DPACS2004 in several ways. The student was directly in charge for this, and in this chapter all the architectural choices will be reported. For the initial paragraph, about O3-DPACS architectural solutions, they have been presented partially in [38], [39], [40].

Under the shell, O3-DPACS behaves as a layered system as DPACS2004 did, so taking full advantage of Java technology, by empowering the portability of Java and the scalability of J2EE application servers.

Whatever the operating system, O3-DPACS relies on a J2EE compatible application server, which is based on the JVM (Java Virtual Machine). The Java layer allows the access to Windows or Linux file-systems. Moreover, using the JDBC interface, the system is also compatible with all the DBMSs, which provide a JDBC driver.

[38] *P. Inchingolo, M. Beltrame, P. Bosazzi, D. Cicuta, G. Faustini, S. Mininel, A. Poli, F. Vatta, O3-DPACS Open-Source Image-Data Manager/Archiver and HDW2 Image-Data Display: An IHE-compliant project pushing the e-health integration in the world. Computerized Medical Imaging and Graphics, Volume 30, Issue 6-7, Pages 391-406*

[39] *Paolo Inchingolo, Marco Beltrame, Pierpaolo Bosazzi, Davide Cicuta, Giorgio Faustini, Andrea Poli, Federica Vatta, The O3-DPACS Open-Source Image-Data Manager/Archiver: a Java-Based, IHE compliant project fostering the e-health integration in the Enlarged Europe, proceed of the 29th ICT International Convention MIPRO 2006, Opatja (Croatia), May 22-26, 2006, vol. 5 (2006)*

[40] *M. Beltrame, P. Bosazzi, A. Poli, P. Inchingolo O3-DPACS: a Java-based, IHE compliant open-source data and image manager and archiver, IFMBE Proceedings MEDICON 2007, "11th Mediterranean Conference on Medical and Biological Engineering and Computing", IFMBE Proceedings Series (ISSN:1680-0737), 2007, Ljubljana, Slovenia, CD.*

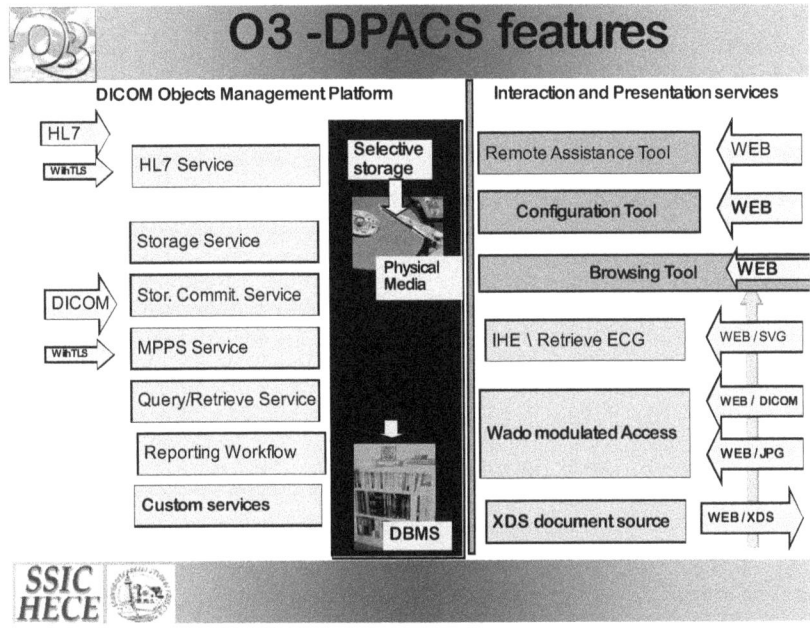

19: O3-DPACS modules and features

Several services were implemented: DICOM Storage, DICOM Modality Performed Procedure Step (MPPS), DICOM Query, DICOM Retrieve, DICOM Storage-Commitment, DICOM reporting workflow and HL7 server. These servers are responsible for receiving a message and understanding whether it is under their responsibility. If so, they call for business logic. It is important to notice that all the servers (either DICOM or HL7) implement either the normal mode or the secure mode through the TLS protocol, where certificates need to be declared.

All the business logic can be invoked by RMI (Remote Method Calls) calls or by other protocols, like web, web services, WADO etc. As a matter of fact a layer for managing DICOM objects (not only images) was created, on the top of it the services can use the layer and translate the data to any protocol. The details are explained later in the project architecture section.

An example of this modular structure and data access is the access to waveform (usually ECG) data. They are stored in DICOM as a normal DICOM store, but the retrieval can be done through two services: the DICOM retrieve or the HTTP retrieve ECG for display, where an SVG track is being delivered. These two services rely on the same business logic and code, but implement different presentation.

53

Therefore, not only DICOM services were exposed, but special attention has been put in making O3-DPACS a brick for inter-hospital, regional or more wide integration. So a module for XDS-I objects publication has been developed, allowing the PACS system to notify to an XDS registry/repository about all the data it has inside, thus allowing the retrieval from a remote information consumer.

DICOM Services or other configuration parameters, such as communication timeouts, AE-Title filters are published on a secure web page, according to the JMX (Java Management eXtensions) standard specifications. Hence, operators can change the configuration from a web page without restarting the system and multiple authentication methods can be implemented to avoid misuse of this critical feature. This is critical since several runtime observations and operations are needed on always running server as the PACS is.

O3-DPACS software structure

20: The O3-DPACS core structure

For managing the services, each logical "server" is bound to an MBean, which is responsible for exposing the methods to change its parameters. In this way, every parameters, in the presentation and communication layer, can be monitored or altered. This structure needs an MBean server to be hosted and solving how this can be done across different application servers is the key to portability as described in next paragraph.

The business logic is written as an Enterprise Java Beans (EJB) layer and its main concern is updating the database, eventually storing data on the file-system and doing additional tasks, thus managing the DICOM objects.

The Java Beans architecture achieves two goals. It fosters scalability since objects are accessed either from local or remote interfaces, that for example could be a requisite to distribute the system on a cluster. Moreover, the EJB interfaces can be easily called from web, via a normal web access, as well as via other applications implementing JNDI (Java Naming and Directory Interface) or RMI (Java Remote Method Invocation); alternatively, they can be used as a web service, again either from an application or from a browser. The dealers serve as a layered structure managing DICOM object. The dealers access the database through JDBC methods; routing to a data-source is defined externally in some deployment descriptors of the application server. This makes it easy to switch between Dbases without altering the application code and constitutes the data-managing layer.

O3 Consortium team chose to use IHE profiles still in the design phase of its products considering it one of the most effective ways to obtain meaningful interoperability. Beside this, several choices have been made in 2007 to make O3-DPACS the best software satisfying the "requirements" and optimally fitting the O3 development and assistance model. Before analyzing one by one these choices, focusing on the most original ones, the IHE integration statement is provided.

Connectathon Europe 2005 and 2006	Key Image Note	Evidence Documents	Reporting Workflow		Consistent Time	Audit Trail and Node Authentication		XDS	XDS for imaging	Scheduled Workflow	Patient Reconciliation (PIR)
	Image Manager	Image Manager	Image Manager	Report Manager	Time Client	Audit Record Repository	Secure Node	Document Source	Imaging Document Source	Image Manager	Image Manager

21: **IHE profiles implemented in O3-DPACS**

55

4.2: Portability

Trying to comply with all the O3 "requirements", a first focus was on the portability. The work done on this topic was presented to EuroPACS [41].

DPACS2004 was already portable on several database management systems (Postgres, MySql) as on different Operating Systems (Windows, Linux). O3-DPACS proved to be portable also on Mac OS-X and,as verified by experimentation, it is portable on different Application Servers. O3-DPACS structure is being re-organized to have it's own MBean Server created on every Application Server leveraging JMX standard Java API. On this element, the business logic elements of the application are registered and the application now can be run on JBOSS AS and SUN AS (Glassfish project) without modifications.

The portability requirement imply the chance to let customer personnel completely choose the platform to use and take the most from internal skills, to reduce costs and increase system reliability. It can be argued that, theoretically, writing an application using Java Enterprise Edition should imply total portability on Application Servers. The response is that: first, it was not evident that a PACS could be written in a totally portable way with good reliability and performance, second, no analogue effort has been reported either as PACS either as other medical system.

The details: the structure of DPACS2004 regarding the use of JMX technology is depicted in the figure:

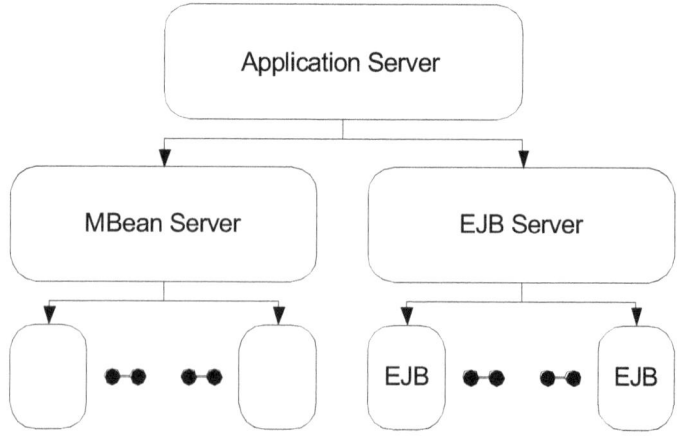

[41] Beltrame M, Ambrogi F, Bosazzi P, Carrara A, Frescura P, Poli A, A new support model for open source critical systems in healthcare: the O3-DPACS experience, submitted to EuroPACS 2008

The MBean server relied on Application Server specific implementation, schema inherited from dcm4jboss that was the inspiration for DPACS2004 version. In that case the application server was JBOSS 3.0.8 and several limitations were present in the model. The implementation of JMX was not the same on all the application servers; the specification for JMX services included in J2EE 1.4 was more focused on server management than on application runtime management and fully included in JBoss 3.08 neither in the 2004 version of SUN application server, and the MBean server implementation was lacking. Moreover, the implementation of JBOSS allowed MBeans to be registered at runtime while JMX original specification at that time did not. This meant that for the SUN reference implementation you had to make coincide the application server lifecycle with your managed application one.

The way to avoid the incompatibility of the MBean server application and allow the same managed services on any platform is to insert a layer of compatibility based on the EJB container.

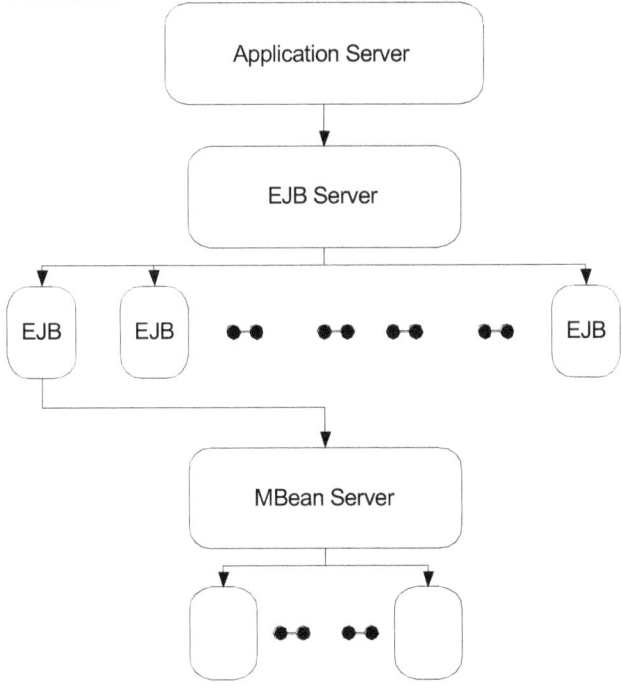

23: The JMX use in O3-DPACS

This allows to use only standard interface towards the application server, to avoid any problem about the start of the MBean server and the registration of the beans and to use an implementation of JMX Mbean included in the application package, implementing the needed classes such as the standard MBean server.

Moreover, the use of EJB as a support for the MBean server allows the use of JNDI to refer to the MBean server. This avoids the use of a common variable reference to the MBean instance, as used in DPACS2004, which was against Java Enterprise specifications.

Once this structure was applied this effort came to face little collateral problems:

- SAAJ implementation: the different implementation of SAAJ, the API for attaching file to SOAP message caused several failure in the building of the message for the publication of images to XDS repository. A little variation in defining the message fragment cause unrecoverable error in the destination message parser (not in Java) and in the official reference implementation.

- Log implementation: every application server (at least SUN's and JBOSS) use a different logging system. It's mandatory to take advantage of Application Server logging infrastructure since it lets the developer forget file rolling, backup and other valuable routines. What it's difficult to obtain, without configuring your own logging environment is to mix your log in the application server one to take advantage of the server navigation tools, such as level browsing and search engines. At the moment O3-DPACS logs?? into the server log on Glassfish and JBOSS but it has issue on Glassfish about?? the understanding of log levels.

Besides these problems, O3-DPACS portability today is a experimented result. The same application is currently servicing three major Italian hospitals: Cattinara Hospital in Trieste, Santa Chiara and Cisanello Hospitals in Pisa and Azienda Ospedaliera in Padova. The first two installations are shifting from production to scientific installation due to regional commercial choices, but still managing the 70% of the total ordinary produced data. Cattinara installation is based on Linux/MySql/Glassfish, Pisa installation on Windows/Postgres/Jboss while Padua installation on Linux Enterprise/MySql/JBoss.

O3-DPACS scalability went also through live tests. Cattinara scientific installation, managing 30.000 studies each year, works with good performance on a simple PC using an AMD Athlon XP 3000+, 2 GB RAM and firewire connected 2 TB storage, while Padua hospital production installation runs on a virtual machine on professional virtualization hardware managing 120.000 exams per year and three levels of storage using all modern storage technologies (NAS, CAS, SUN).

Good performances means that from user perspective a query against current day exams should last less then 5 second and the time for retrieving an exam should remain in the order of the network transfer time. Obviously, to be referred as good performances, they should remain stable on the long period and do not degrade in a significant way.

It must be said that the solution designed is today working and allows the personalization of the monitoring services either on the web (look and feel) either in the code development but, from the time of research and design, several alternatives would be worth to be evaluated in the future. By example, JMX today allows listing the Mbean servers in the current application server and choosing the suitable one to register your Mbean, or to create your own with a label, recalling it by that label instead of via JNDI and remote interfaces. This method may be more efficient and less code consuming. Anyway, what is not foreseen as solved is the way to register the Mbean at runtime, letting you stop, start and add monitored services in your Mbean server instance. At the moment, no other methods but the supporting EJB for managing the Mbean server lifecycle has been positively evaluated.

4.3: Project design issues

Another original contribution by the student was the O3-DPACS project design[42], which had the goals to:

- fit the O3 development model
- maximize the management of code reliability
- maximize external contributions thus reducing the invested resources

A premise is recalling the existence of the O3 Consortium website where downloads and collaborative tools, such as CVS and support and discussion forums are available to user, completing a simple registration. It is extremely valuable for monitoring the trend of interest, market and research requests, and involve the downloader into online discussion.

To make a critical system live in the online community environment, and recalling the discussion about requirements in the previous paragraphs, the challenge was to design a software project that:

- should persist and manage data in an open format, decreasing to zero the chance to have difficulties during the data access even in case of failure or extreme emergency

- should reach the balance between the need to limit modifications across versions, in order to maintain stress-tested reliability, and the need to

---

[42] Beltrame M, Bosazzi P, Carrara A, Poli A, O3-DPACS system: challenges and original solutions in developing an open source project for the PACS critical system, accepted to euroPACS 2008.

develop continuous modification to stay on the edge and beyond, as it's vital being O3 natively a research project

- should ease the collaborative work and the maintenance of the code

- should fit perfectly the O3 development model

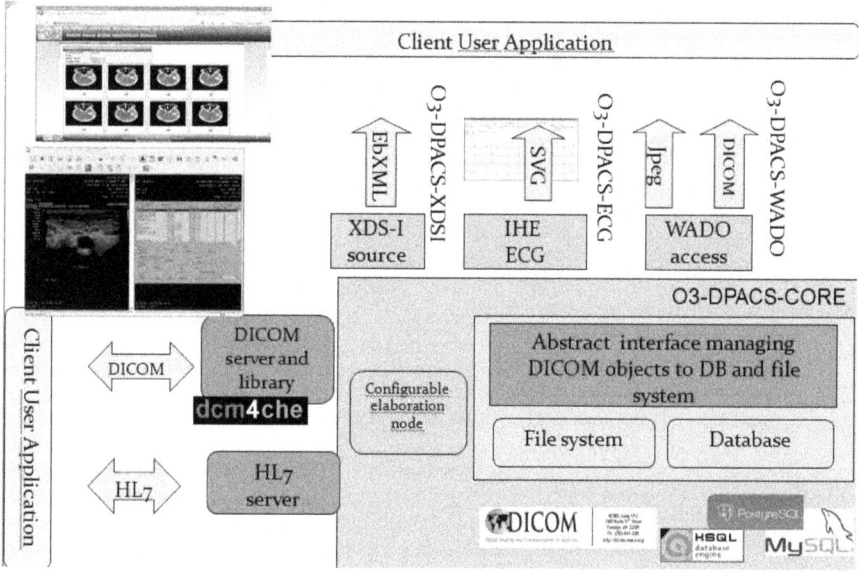

24: O3-DPACS project structure

To achieve such goals O3-DPACS project was divided logically in two sections (picture 22): an *"engine"* layer managing DICOM objects and a *"presentation layer"* for communication of those objects. At the same time, the project was divided as several development projects, a *"core"* project and some *"presentation"* projects that can or cannot be packed with the core project.

Two choices were done for the core project. One is storing the original DICOM data as it came out from the source. This was mainly due to two reasons: the first is letting data be accessible even if the software goes down, the second is that no software should alter the original data, which is considered as *"the document"*. The second choice is to build a layer of software that can hide the managing of DICOM objects to applications. The layer is built into the core as a collection of Java

60

Enterprise Bean, which can be asked from local or remote application to save or return information about DICOM entities. DICOM is today increasing its capacity to describe different kinds of data, and O3-DPACS can include images, reports, evidences, waveforms, multiframes and documents.

The presentation layer projects have been created to give access to DICOM data using the appropriate way for each real world application. ECG module presents ECGs from DICOM in SVG vectorial format, adhering to the IHE Retrieve ECG for display profile. The WADO module presents DICOM in JPEG with requested dimensions and quality via WEB. The XDS-I module can export data to an XDS-I Repository to share O3-DPACS data in an Electronic Health Record. All these modules, including the DICOM communication module implemented on top of DCM4CHE libraries, call for the same methods into the core project to get data.

We recall that reliability is the main requirement, and for a PACS it means that it must, at any time, allow the visualization and creation of a report for an emergency exam, in a filmless environment. The proposed design implies several advantages for reliability. On one side, the core project can easily be kept under the control of O3 core development team and be finely tuned according to production experience. Moreover, applications that take advantage of core methods implicitly use the auditing and logging routines built into the core, leading to the traceability of every use of sensible information, and thus increasing security. At the same time, the community can freely contribute to all the other modules without impact to the reliability of the core project and make the project be fed by its driving force.

4.4: Other original aspects

4.4. 1: Performance preview

A collateral result regarding performance was obtained during experimentation. The performance of series preview on the DICOM viewer was addressed. O3 radiology workstation O3-RWS[43] lets browse series once the user has selected an exam to view. It's a common feature in commercial workstations too. Usually this is done downloading via DICOM, or in a faster proprietary way, one image from the series.

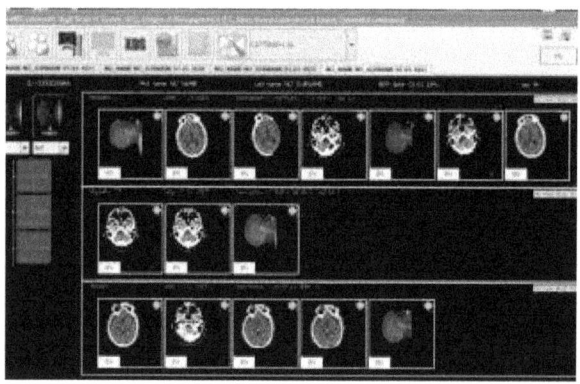

25: Effect of O3-RWS use of WADO for the preview

We propose to do it via WADO services, as we noted that the most of modern PACS implement this standard DICOM service. The viewer, when showing the preview of the series, should ask the configured PACS for a JPEG image of reduced dimensions as a thumbnail for the preview. Such a procedure has several advantages: optimize transfer time of the preview, since low quality is enough for this purpose, let the viewer ask for the needed dimensions and, most important, a viewer from any vendor would be able to ask for a thumbnail to a PACS from any vendor but implementing WADO. The procedure is being considered to be proposed to IHE committee as an option for scheduled workflow profile.

---

[43] Faustini, Poli, Inchingolo, O3-RWS: a Java-based, IHE-compliant open-source radiology workstation, IFMBE Proceedings MEDICON 2007, "11th Mediterranean Conference on Medical and Biological Engineering and Computing", IFMBE Proceedings Series (ISSN:1680-0737), 2007, Ljubljana, Slovenia, CD.

4.4.2: Database performance and common open source adoption behavior

Today PACS applications struggle on two performance indicators: the time to respond to a query and the time for the retrieval of images. They are the two times when the user is waiting on the screen, and therefore can state ""it's slow. Storing, by example, usually goes on background and cannot be stated if it's fast enough unless you stop with a chronometer on the modality console.

It was demonstrated that during a query, the time consumption of the code is negligible in comparison with the time the DMBS uses to respond to the query. So in a query, the DBMS (or the way it is used) is the responsible for performance. In the production environment of Padua the Postgres DBMS 7.4 suffered from 100% decay of performance on a test query in one month, after a year of work and database loading.

The query was asking for "all the exam of a predetermined day" and the decay was evaluated being caused by the type of engine Postgres uses, associated by the common use of default configuration.

It is indeed a common situation when you, service deliverer, don't have an experienced assistant on every open source component you are going to let the customer choose, unless you have an advised suite on which your experts are particular competent. That's a consequence of the liberty of choice that is permitted to customer but it's also a collateral reason to take advantage of internal customer knowledge as discussed about the support model sustainability.

Therefore, unless the customer chooses the recommended software stack from O3, where the expertise on the systemistic and database level is excellent, you don't expect anyone in the installation would go far beyond default configuration of the DBMS, as it is for application server, virtual machine and so on.

Anyway, Postgres provides tools that take the situation back to optimal performance, but causes slowness during maintenance execution or needs to stop the DBMS. While several combination of the use of the Vacuum tool was tested, the problem could not be taken to zero impact. We refer to Postgres 8.0, as 8.1 was out only later, and has an *autovacuum* daemon that could not be tested in the production environment.

The reason for this behavior being unacceptable is that the implementation of the system is in a 24h a day running environment, as the healthcare applications like PACS are. In this environment, the slowness or stop for *vaccuming* cuts down the service uptime at acceptable performance to unacceptable level for the support contracts. Simulations on Postgres 8.1 and the *autovaccum* daemon did not resolve the problem, even if the load could not be replicated in 1:1 scale, and neither the documentation nor literature helped. Moreover, some limitations are known: it pays no attention to how much busy the server is: there were plans to check system load before vacuuming, but that's not a current feature. So if you have extreme load peaks, *autovacuum* may not be suitable for your installation.

Anyway, no one in the literature would say Postgres is better or worse than any other database, recalling that it depends on the use you do of it.

Then, since it's known from literature that query performance against a Postgres database decay when updates are done on the DB, caused most probably by the persisting of old rows in the file system, a choice was trying to use a different DBMS.

The choice was using MySql 5. The migration of data was done with a script produced in a day, thanks to the open source and standard stack of both DBMS. After four months of production runtime, the new DBMS showed increased performances in query e no decay in performance on the test query (<5%).

Since O3-DPACS doesn't use any native feature of the DBMS, Postgres seems less suiting a critical 24h/24h 7/7d system than MySql, using default configuration and the provided tools as in a typical open source application. This is the reason because from 2007 MySql is recommended for the use with O3-DPACS.

Conclusions

The personal research project conducted by the PhD student was inserted in the O3 Consortium research project, with the aim to propose a complete solution for the adoption of open technology in the healthcare environment.

The PhD student contributed in thinking and designing all the aspects of the complete solution presented in this thesis, in the development and business models as well as in developing the products and in writing and publishing the results of this team work.

He personally contributed to the model with the original idea of the support model and with the design and main implementation of a product to test the proposed ideas

The student had an intermediate step in his personal project: to built a state of the art server for the management of DICOM objects, with the aim to ease the adoption of e-health technology and to develop a product on which the model would have been tested. The research was conducted in the following way: first, the definition of O3 Consortium project software design guidelines was performed, through an analysis of real world needs, literature and past experience. They were called "requirements" in the thesis, then the product was designed and developed implementing original solutions to best achieve all those "requirements". The technological choices and the original aspects against the state of the art have been discussed and underlined throughout all the thesis, such as the compliance to all the requirements and the choices for portability, project organization, standard implementation and performance, while the idea of O3-DPACS being an integrated project, system plus support model, have been discussed. It should be remarked again that O3 Consortium means not only software development but also new procedures in technology delivering and service delivering over technology.

The student believes to have put strong basis for the project to remain on the edge of technology and for the research and proposal of new models. Moreover, he concluded the validation of the software and the model, which was needed to verify the assumption and to obtain the first results in O3 Consortium research on *e-health* adoption.

Should be reminded that O3 Consortium project peculiarity of proposing a whole complete application model to the healthcare real world of open source software is an original effort. No other solution for open source software application makes a complete proposal for all the topics of development, design, software architecture and support. Thus, a real research interest exists in testing and validating the model.

Future work for the aims of the project would concern following the technology evolution, the reporting automation problem and the clinical data integration in wide areas such as regions. First, technology is always running: this year new DICOM classes describing the last data intensive acquisition modalities have been included into the standard. IHE basic profiles like Scheduled Workflow are going under review and Java Enterprise Edition is coming to Edition 5, sliding to web service and providing different and more efficient methods to go to databases. This technological evolution should be addressed and it is not only a matter of rewriting the code. For example, the new DICOM CT classes incorporates in a DICOM file more than one images and therefore it implies to change what is to be considered atomic in the database and in the PACS system.

The second aspect is the reporting workflow automation. In Italy but also in Europe a way to assign efficiently the exam to review to the radiologist or the reporting physician is requested. An even harder request is from tele-radiology and tele-medicine centers that request for the generation of the work list for their tasks. IHE has a profile for this but is lacking on task assignment and work list generation methods. That should be addressed in this year.

Last, the PACS system should be only a brick in the electronic health record of the citizen, recalling DPACS project and O3 Consortium project mission. O3-DPACS has been extended to do it, but the whole system should be tuned. The infrastructure is mostly ready (IHE XDS plus extensions) but semantical interoperability relies on organization and users choices that should be analyzed and discussed. The student did a study[44] on the whole electronic health record system integration with mobile device, a study and design should be done for regional whole clinical data integration using O3 design guidelines.

As a conclusion, O3-DPACS integrated system, made of the product and the support model, is a personal original proposal in the new complete solution called O3 Consortium project. A battle-field validation of the O3 Consortium statements has been conducted, beyond the proposal to the academic literature, and the goals of the project seem to be reachable. Last, the outcome of this research is patrimony also of O3-Enterprise, that would apply the discussed ideas to the market. Its successful creation, joining the support of the University and a major industrial partner, is yet another proof of the potential of these outcomes.

---

[44] Progetto D4, Progetto di sviluppo tecnologico: Sviluppo di strumenti di interoperabilità per l'integrazione tra strutture sanitarie e cittadino con particolare riguardo al contesto del FVG, Assegnista: ing. Marco Beltrame, R. Sc.: Prof. Paolo Inchingolo, R. Az. Ing. Massimo Piccinin.

Bibliography

Inchingolo P, Beltrame M, Bosazzi P, Cicuta D, Faustini G, Mininel S, Poli A, Vatta F, O3-DPACS Open-Source Image-Data Manager/Archiver and HDW2 Image-Data Display: An IHE-compliant project pushing the e-health integration in the world (2006), Computerized Medical Imaging and Graphics, 30(6-7):391-406

2

M. Diminich, P. Inchingolo, F. Magliacca and N. Martinolli, Versatile and open tools for LAN, MAN and WAN communications with PACS. In: K.D. Held, C.A. Brebbia, R.D. Ciskowski and H. Power, Editors, Computational biomedicine, Computational Mechanics Publications, Southampton (1993), pp. 309–316

3

P. Inchingolo, From the GNBTS-NET to the biomedical communication network of Trieste. In: M. Bracale and F. Denoth, Editors, Proceedings of the MEDICON '92, Area di Ricerca, CNR, Pisa (1992), pp. 1239–1242.

4

M. Diminich, P. Inchingolo, N. Martinolli, L. Dalla Palma, P. Giribona and R. Pozzi et al., ARIS: an autonomous remote image station offering both local and remote IMACS/RIS resources in an open environment, Proceedings of the Third European Conference on Engineering Medicine (1995), p. 241

5

F. Fioravanti, P. Inchingolo, G. Valenzin, L. Dalla Palma and R. Vallon, The DPACS Project at the University of Trieste: architecture and working environment, Proceedeedings of the 14th International EuroPACS Meeeting Creta, Greece (1996).

6

F. Fioravanti, P. Inchingolo, G. Valenzin, L. Dalla Palma and R. Vallon, HIS-RIS-PACS integration with the DPACS Project at the University of Trieste, Proceedings of the 14th International EuroPACS Meeeting Creta, Greece (1996).

7

F. Fioravanti, P. Inchingolo, G. Valenzin and P.L. Dalla, The DPACS Project at the University of Trieste, Med Informat **22** (1997) (4), pp. 301–314

8

P. Inchingolo, Trieste and Region Friuli-Venezia Giulia: an example of fully-managed health telematics system the new Telematic Network of 2000's Trieste, IFMBE Proceedings **1** (2001), pp. 78–81.

9

Europacs 2004, www.tbs.ts.it/europacs2004

0

Integrating the Healthcare Enterprise web site, www.ihe.net

1

MARIS project home: http://maris.homelinux.org

2

Inchingolo P, Londero F, Vatta F, The E-HECE e-Learning Experience in BME Education (2007) in: IFMBE Proceedings MEDICON 2007, "11th Mediterranean Conference on Medical and Biological Engineering and Computing", IFMBE Proceedings Series (ISSN:1680-0737), 2007, Ljubljana, Slovenia, CD, pp. 1107-1110

3

Higher Education in Clinical Engineering website, http://www.ssic.units.it

4

Fioravanti F, Inchingolo P, Valenzin G, Dalla Palma L, The DPACS project at the University of Trieste (1997), Med Inform (Lond)., 22(4):301-14.

5

Inchingolo P, Picture Archiving and Communications Systems in Today's Healthcare (1997), WMA Journal (WMJ)

6 Imaging management journal web page, http://www.imagingmanagement.org/

7

A. T. Bui. & Kangarloo, H. (2005), 'openSourcePACS: An extensible infrastructure for medical image management', IEEE TRANSACTIONS ON INFORMATION TECHNOLOGY IN BIOMEDICINE, TITB-00168-2005.R1.

8

DCM4CHE project, www.dcm4che.org

9

Norio Nakata, Yasushi Fukuda, Kunihiko Fukuda and Naoki Suzuki, DICOM Wiki: Web-based collaboration and knowledge database system for radiologists, International Congress Series, Volume 1281, CARS 2005: Computer Assisted Radiology and Surgery, May 2005, Pages 980-985.

20

Norio Nakata, Yasushi Fukuda, Kunihiko Fukuda and Naoki Suzuki, DICOM Wiki: Web-based collaboration and knowledge database system for radiologists, International Congress Series, Volume 1281, CARS 2005: Computer Assisted Radiology and Surgery, May 2005, Pages 980-985

2

de Regt, David, Weinberger, Ed, MyFreePACS: A Free Web-Based Radiology Image Storage and Viewing   Tool
Am. J. Roentgenol. 2004 183: 535-537

22

Cuadros J, Sim I. EyePACS: an open source clinical communication system for eye care. Medinfo 2004;11:207-11

23

Puech PA, Boussel L, Belfkih S, Lemaitre L, Douek P, Beuscart R., DicomWorks: software for reviewing DICOM studies and promoting low-cost teleradiology, J Digit Imaging., 2007 Jun;20(2):122-30

24

Marcheschi, P.; Positano, V.; Ferdeghini, E.M.; Mazzarisi, A.; Benassi, A., "An open source based application for integration and sharing of multi-modal cardiac image data in a heterogeneous environment," Computers in Cardiology, 2003 , vol., no., pp. 367-370, 21-24 Sept. 2003

25

Inchingolo P., Bosazzi P., Cicuta D., Faustini G., Barbaro A., Vittor A. Miniussi E., DPACS-2004 becomes a java-based open-source modular system in proceedings of EUROPACS-MIR, 2004

26

Lakovidis, I.; Pattichis, C.S.; Schizas, C.N., "Guest Editorial Special Issue on Emerging Health Telematics Applications in Europe," Information Technology in Biomedicine, IEEE Transactions on , vol.2, no.3, pp.110-116, Sep 1998

27

Istepanian, R.S.H.; Jovanov, E.; Zhang, Y.T., "Guest Editorial Introduction to the Special Section on M-Health: Beyond Seamless Mobility and Global Wireless Health-Care Connectivity," Information Technology in Biomedicine, IEEE Transactions on , vol.8, no.4, pp. 405-414, Dec. 2004

28

Grimes, S.L., "The challenge of integrating the healthcare enterprise," Engineering in Medicine and Biology Magazine, IEEE , vol.24, no.2, pp. 122-124, March-April 2005

29

 Joomla, content manager system, http://www.joomla.org/

30

Beltrame M, Ambrogi F, Bosazzi P, Carrara A, Frescura F, Poli A, A new support model for open source critical systems in healthcare: the O3-DPACS experience, submitted to EuroPACS 2008.

3

Ratib O, Swiernik M, McCoy JM, From PACS to integrated EMR (2003), Computerized Medical Imaging and Graphics, 27(2-3):207-215.

32

Dinevski D, Inchingolo P, Krajnc I, Kokol P, "Open Source Software in Health Care and Open Three Example" (2007), Computer-Based Medical Systems, 2007. CBMS '07. Twentieth IEEE International Symposium on , pp.33-40, 20-22 June 2007

33

Bui AT, Kangarloo H., 'openSourcePACS: An extensible infrastructure for medical image management' (2005), IEEE TRANSACTIONS ON INFORMATION TECHNOLOGY IN BIOMEDICINE, TITB-00168-2005.R1.

34

Marcheschi P, Positano V, Ferdeghini EM, Mazzarisi A, Benassi A, "An open source based application for integration and sharing of multi-modal cardiac image data in a heterogeneous environment" (2003), Computers in Cardiology, 367-370

35

McDonald CJ, Schadow G, Barnes M, Dexter P, Overhage JM, Mamlin B, McCoy JM, Open Source software in medical informatics--why, how and what, (2003), International Journal of Medical Informatics, 69(2-3):175-184.

36

Zhao L and Elbaum S, Quality assurance under the open source development model, Journal of Systems and Software, 66(1):65-75.

37

Ratib O and Rosset A, Open-source software in medical imaging: development of OsiriX (2006), International Journal of Computer Assisted Radiology and Surgery, 1(4):187-196

38

P. Inchingolo, M. Beltrame, P. Bosazzi, D. Cicuta, G. Faustini, S. Mininel, A. Poli, F. Vatta, O3-DPACS Open-Source Image-Data Manager/Archiver and HDW2 Image-Data Display: An IHE-compliant project pushing the e-health integration in the world. Computerized Medical Imaging and Graphics, Volume 30, Issue 6-7, Pages 391-406

39

Paolo Inchingolo, Marco Beltrame, Pierpaolo Bosazzi, Davide Cicuta, Giorgio Faustini, Andrea Poli, Federica Vatta, The O3-DPACS Open-Source Image-Data Manager/Archiver: a Java-Based, IHE compliant project fostering the e-health integration in the Enlarged Europe, proceed of the 29th ICT International Convention MIPRO 2006, Opatja (Croatia), May 22-26, 2006, vol. 5 (2006)

40

M. Beltrame, P. Bosazzi, A. Poli, P. Inchingolo O3-DPACS: a Java-based, IHE compliant open-source data and image manager and archiver, IFMBE Proceedings MEDICON 2007, "11th Mediterranean Conference on Medical and Biological Engineering and Computing", IFMBE Proceedings Series (ISSN:1680-0737), 2007, Ljubljana, Slovenia, CD.

4

Beltrame M, Ambrogi F, Bosazzi P, Carrara A, Frescura P, Poli A, A new support model for open source critical systems in healthcare: the O3-DPACS experience, accepted to EuroPACS 2008

42

Beltrame M, Bosazzi P, Carrara A, Poli A, O3-DPACS system: challenges and original solutions in developing an open source project for the PACS critical system, accepted to euroPACS 2008.

43

Faustini, Poli, Inchingolo, O3-RWS: a Java-based, IHE-compliant open-source radiology workstation, IFMBE Proceedings MEDICON 2007, "11th Mediterranean Conference on Medical and Biological Engineering and Computing", IFMBE Proceedings Series (ISSN:1680-0737), 2007, Ljubljana, Slovenia, CD.

44

Progetto D4, Progetto di sviluppo tecnologico: Sviluppo di strumenti di interoperabilità per l'integrazione tra strutture sanitarie e cittadino con particolare riguardo al contesto del FVG, Assegnista: ing. Marco Beltrame, R. Sc.: Prof. Paolo Inchingolo, R. Az. Ing. Massimo Piccinin.

Acknowledgments

This work took three hard years of my life. I went from being graduated to the work of laboratories in some days. Slowly my skill increased as well as the determination of the group in believing that a mark in the e-health world could be written.

It's unbelievable how much I have learnt in these years, technically, but also as human relationship, and personal awareness. It's unbelievable how much I pushed myself on this project and how, more than sometimes, I suffered for it. It's unbelievable how many times I had the feeling that a great event could happen with a really little effort more...and it didn't. It's unbelievable how situations could change in months.

Remembering the death of Prof. Paolo Inchingolo, to whom I owe his will of putting his young collaborators in front of the problems, remembering the support that most of the colleagues in Trieste and Padua gave me, in the difficult and the successful times, to whom I owe the many lessons I have learnt, and remembering how much I and my willful colleagues pushed ourselves in it, I felt that this work had to be written, despite the many difficulties I had to pass around in the path of the PhD course.

Many things could have been gone wrong, but this adventure will remain a great richness for me and I think, and hope, for you all that played a role in it.

 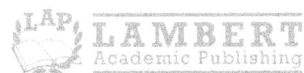 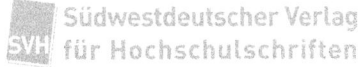

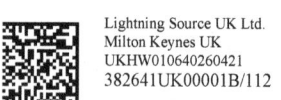

Lightning Source UK Ltd.
Milton Keynes UK
UKHW010640260421
382641UK00001B/112